# TopHealth
## a l m a n a c
### 2001

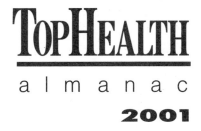

# TopHealth

a l m a n a c

## 2001

Rob Kinslow
Zorba Paster, M.D.
Editors

Renee Zemanski
Contributing Editor

Oakstone Wellness Publishing
Birmingham, Alabama

TopHealth Almanac 2001 is published to provide employees, members of organizations and other readers with the information and motivation needed to achieve and maintain a healthier lifestyle. The content herein is in no way intended as medical advice on individual health problems. Such should be obtained directly from a physician.

To order additional copies of this publication, contact Oakstone Publishing, 6801 Cahaba Valley Road, Birmingham, AL 35242; 800-871-9525

First Printing, August, 2000
ISBN: 0-9675599-1-X
Product Code: 21201
Printed in the United States of America

Publisher: Dennis Hofmaier
Managing Editor: Rhonda Gant Ruiz

Cover design, text design and composition by D. Gardner, Oakstone Publishing
Illustrations by B. Dupree and S. Carter

# about
# TopHealth

First published in 1987, TopHealth is one of the most widely read health and wellness newsletters designed specifically for the workplace. With its focus on illness prevention, self-care and stress management, TopHealth delivers a unique take-charge-of-your-health, take-charge-of-your-life message to more than 2.5 million readers throughout the year.

Award winning and motivational, TopHealth has helped hundreds of organizations trim their bottom lines by encouraging decreased absenteeism and increased productivity. For more information on our family of newsletters, brochures and other TopHealth products, call 800-871-9525.

# t a b l e   o f   c o n t e n t s

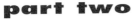

## part one
### A Year of Good Health

There is so much you can do to add years to your life and
quality of life to your years — day in and day out. And it
isn't as hard as you might think. Make way for the 7 Eternal
Laws of Healthy Living.

## part two
### Healthy Living
### Month by Month

January to December, each month presents its own challenges
— as well as numerous opportunities to turn the occasional
good intention into a lifelong habit.

## April

## May

## June

## July

## August

## September

# t a b l e   o f   c o n t e n t s

## part three

You don't have to keep your eye on the calendar
to follow these timeless wellness classics.

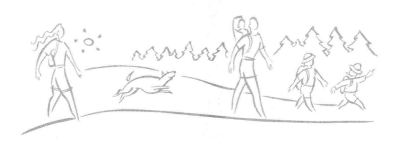

# part four

"The first wealth is health." — Ralph Waldo Emerson

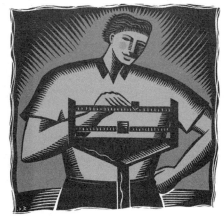

## part one

A Year of
Good Health

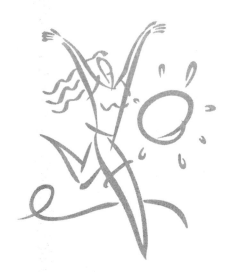

# A Year of
# Good Health

Ready to get started on your healthiest year yet? You've come
to the right place. In these pages you'll find some of the best of
TOPHEALTH — from simple stressbusters to help you cope with
everyday life, to big-picture stuff, such as how to prevent heart
disease and add years to your life.

The TOPHEALTH Almanac is designed to be practical. We've
organized this year's edition month by month, so you can
introduce healthy habits a little at a time — the way experts
say you're most likely to achieve success and form good habits
for life.

Maybe you'd like to get through the winter with fewer colds this
year. Perhaps you'd like to lose a few pounds come spring. Or
maybe you'd just like to inject more fun in your life all year-
round. You'll find it all here: simple, practical, easy-to-follow tips
that can help you feel better, look younger, and yes, live longer.

Ready? To get started, turn the page and read "The 7 Eternal
Laws of Healthy Living." Then use the rest of this book to help
you follow these basic principles of good health. In just a matter
of weeks you'll be on your way to your healthiest year ever — by
December you may declare it your best year yet.

# The 7 Eternal Laws of Healthy Living

Health studies are notorious for saying one thing one day, another thing the next. But these rules of good health never change:

**1** ## Stay physically active.

Find something you love doing in every season — walking in spring, swimming in summer, biking in fall or skiing in winter, for example. Experts say that if it's something you enjoy, you'll stick with it. Just remember that whatever you do, spend at least 30 minutes each day 5 days a week at it. That's how little it takes to reap the health benefits of regular exercise.

**2** ## Eat a healthy diet.

You can't go wrong if you favor "plant" foods, such as whole grains and fresh fruits and vegetables. They're loaded with vitamins, minerals, fiber and other substances like phytochemicals that help your body in countless ways. And when you fill up on plant foods, there's less room for animal fats, which contribute to clogged arteries, and sweets, which can pile on empty calories.

**3** ## Maintain a healthy weight.

Keeping your body trim and avoiding excess weight helps ward off many serious problems, such as heart disease, high blood pressure, diabetes and arthritis. To lose a pound of fat in a week, remember another immutable law, **the 500 Rule:** To lose that pound, you need to consume an average 500 calories less or burn 500 more per day than you already do to maintain your current weight.

**4** ## Don't use any form of tobacco.

Smoking causes nearly one in five deaths in the United States and shortens life expectancy by 10-12 years. But even smokeless tobacco hurts: It leads to cancers of the mouth, gum, pharynx, larynx and esophagus. Fact is, snuff dippers consume on average more than 10 times the amount of cancer-causing substances that cigarette smokers do.

## 5 Drink in moderation, if at all.

True, alcohol has heart benefits, but only in small amounts (no more than two drinks in a day for men, one for women). Doctors say that's no reason to take up drinking, however. For one thing, moderate drinking increases the risk of dying from accidents or violence, and habitual drinking can lead to addiction and personal troubles. Besides, there are many wonderful, nonalcoholic ways to help your heart — from upping your fruit and vegetable intake to taking a daily walk with a friend.

## 6 Always think safety first.

Some accidents are simply bad luck, but the truth is that most can be prevented, so don't take unnecessary risks — with your health or your life. Use seat belts and car safety seats ... wear protective equipment at work if your job requires it ... use the right gear at home when working with power tools or hazardous chemicals.

## 7 See your doctor regularly for preventive care.

See your doctor regularly for preventive care. Screening tests — like mammograms and blood cholesterol and blood pressure checks — can detect many diseases in their early stages when they may be more successfully treated. Talk to your physician about what tests you need and how often they should be performed.

Follow these tips, and you'll discover that you have more energy, less worry, and years of happiness to look forward to. Not bad for just seven little steps, eh?

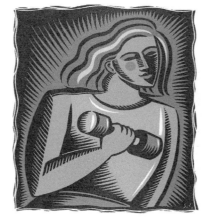

part two

## Healthy Living
## Month by Month

# Healthy Living
# Month by Month

January to December, each month presents its own challenges — as well as numerous opportunities to turn the occasional good intention into a lifelong habit.

# January

Named for Janus, the Roman god of new beginnings, this is the month for a fresh start on the road to better health. It's also a time to avoid cold-weather maladies such as the common cold.

## Your Healthiest
## Year Ever

The New Year can be a great opportunity to start fresh. And New Year's **resolutions** can be a powerful tool to give your health a big boost and improve your whole life. Far too often, though, resolutions don't last past February or March. Instead of motivating you for success, resolutions are often unrealistic — and can make you feel like you've failed.

Why are so many resolutions abandoned so early? Most often it's because people set their goals too high — and don't have a clear battle plan on how to get there. What to do? As with any project, at work or around the house, the key to success is to decide on a series of achievable action steps — with target dates attached.

## "I'll get more exercise."

**Action steps:** "Because I'm over 40 and I've been inactive, first I'll check with my doctor before starting my fitness program. Then I'll take advantage of the special rates offered at my local fitness center and join by the first week in January. I'll try to go to the center once a week for the first month, twice a week the second month and then three times a week. In the spring, I'll start taking lunch-hour walks with a co-worker."

## "I'll eat less fat."

**Action steps:** "I'll go easy on high-fat sweets beginning right now. Then I'll start choosing a baked potato (hold the sour cream) instead of fries at the cafeteria. By March, I'll start introducing my whole family to the idea of snacking on pretzels and fruit instead of potato chips and candy. In June, I'll reward myself with a weekly treat of yogurt ice cream and start a collection of my favorite low-fat recipes."

## "I'll drink less alcohol."

**Action steps:** "If I drink on a regular basis, I'll gradually work my way down to just a drink or two a day, tops. And even if I only drink occasionally at parties, I'll always quit after two drinks — and I won't drink at all if I'm a designated driver."

**The bottom line:** Wars are won battle by battle, and no resolution was ever worth making if it didn't have a smart action plan.

# Resolution Hints

- Start now by focusing on one or two unhealthy habits that may be trouble spots in your lifestyle.

- Next, think of all the better alternatives that you could substitute.

- Then, decide how best to begin making changes, starting gradually and working onward and upward.

- Share your plan with friends, family, and co-workers — and try to enlist a "buddy" to make changes with you and keep you honest.

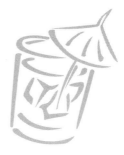

# Winning the Cold Wars

Yes, it's true: We've landed on the moon, but we still don't have a cure for the common cold. This pesky ailment is the most common health reason for lost days from work. At least 200 different viruses can cause colds. That's why it's been so hard to develop a vaccine against them.

If your luck is average, the odds are you'll get two or three colds this year. How will you ease your discomfort, scratchy throat, runny nose, coughing and sneezing?

## Go with the Proven Solutions

Enjoy a long steamy shower. Avoid tobacco smoke, and drink plenty of fluids like water, juice, tea and soup. These liquids help loosen stuffiness in the sinuses and chest. And, research at Harvard Medical School, UCLA and Mount Sinai Medical Center support that chicken soup really does relieve cold symptoms, especially congestion.

## Choose the Right Weapon

If any symptom is especially distressing to you during the course of your cold, aim a single targeted treatment at it. **Example:** Try acetaminophen (like Tylenol) for fever and muscle aches; a decongestant like pseudoephedrine (such as Sudafed) for a stuffy nose; a cough expectorant like guaifenesin (Robitussin) for a dry, unproductive cough; or a cough suppressant like dextromethorphan (Pertussin) at night if coughing is keeping you awake.

### What about zinc?

Some studies have shown zinc lozenges to reduce length and severity of colds, while others have shown no benefit. Because the jury is still out, essentially, it's best to check with your doctor about trying zinc to fight a cold.

## What NOT to Take

For colds, researchers warn against taking antihistamines, which can worsen symptoms. And they question the "shotgun" approach of the many combination cold products on which we spend over a billion dollars a year. These products, which contain several drugs mixed together, can cause unwanted side effects, while not delivering enough of whatever ingredient you actually need most at the time.

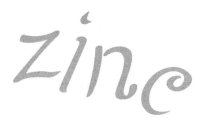

## When to Seek Help

There's rarely a need to see a doctor for a cold because colds nearly always go away on their own within 10 days. But if you have cold-like symptoms for more than two weeks (or a fever above 101° for over three days), do call your doctor: Your cold may have evolved into a sinus infection, ear infection, bronchitis — or even pneumonia. These infections are usually caused by bacteria, which require treatment with an antibiotic, like penicillin or erythromycin. In contrast, antibiotics are useless against viruses, including cold viruses.

## Self-Defense

Unlike flu viruses, cold viruses are not as often passed through kissing, coughing or sneezing. And colds are not caused — or even encouraged — by quick changes in weather, sitting in drafts, getting chills, or going out in winter without a hat or with wet hair. The viruses that cause colds are spread most often from the nose to the hand of an infected person, and then from the hand to the nose of a healthy one. So to protect yourself …

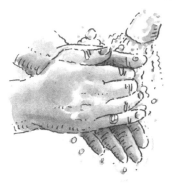

- **Wash your hands often.**

- **Keep your hands away from your face.**

# 4 Winter Tips
# for Your Health
# & Safety

If you plan to travel where there's chilly
weather or if you live in a cold climate,
keep these safety tips in mind:

**1** On the road.

Use your low beam headlights when dri-
ving through fog or snowstorms — they'll actually provide better visi-
bility than high beams. And be prepared for breakdowns with emergency flares, warm blanket, first-aid kit, white cloth to
signal distress, flashlight, snow shovel, empty gas can, and, for long
trips, food and water.

**2** At home.

Carbon monoxide, a colorless, odorless gas and a by-product of com-
bustion, is an invisible killer. **Possible sources include:** wood-burning
stoves, fireplaces, kerosene, gas or oil heaters and furnaces. **For your
protection:** Assure proper ventilation, have these devices inspected
and consider installing carbon monoxide detectors.

**3** Under the sun.

Sunburns aren't limited to summer. Fact is, sunlight in winter can
burn, especially when reflected off ice or snow. So when skiing or
otherwise enjoying the outdoors, wear sunglasses that protect your
eyes against ultraviolet light, and spread sunscreen on exposed skin,
including your lips.

**4** Over exposed.

Watch for frostbite or hypothermia, and seek help without delay if
you suspect either. Danger signs for frostbite ... redness, tingling,
stinging pain or small white patches on the skin ... for hypothermia
... uncontrollable shivering, sleepiness, shallow breathing. **Remember:**
Alcohol increases loss of body heat, so avoid its use when you plan
to be outdoors for a long time.

## Indoor Allergies?

Australian researchers found a simple solution if you're allergic to dust mites and suspect your area rugs make you sneeze and itch: Place the rugs outdoors in direct sunlight for a few hours.

**How it works:** Airing out rugs and other household items dries and heats them — exterminating mites.

# February

Ah, February. The month in which boys' and girls' young hearts first go a-flutter over valentines is also time for American Heart Month, Wise Health Consumer Month, and National Child Passenger Safety Awareness Week.

## How to Avoid a Broken Heart

To protect yourself from heart attacks, first pay attention to how the heart works. Quite simply, your life depends on it. This miraculous pump is actually a specialized muscle the size of your fist that contracts an astounding 100,000 times a day. Each forceful heartbeat helps push your blood through 60,000 miles of blood vessels. The blood brings the 300 trillion-plus cells in your body fresh oxygen and nutrients and carries away the wastes these cells produce.

But the heart too needs plenty of oxygen and nutrients to do its hard job. Special blood vessels called the coronary arteries deliver these valuable supplies to the heart muscle itself. If these arteries become clogged with cholesterol-fat deposits and clots, the flow of supplies is reduced to a trickle and the "starved" heart muscle gets damaged.

# Protecting Your Ticker

Each time you make a heart-healthy choice, you're strengthening your body against a life-threatening emergency. **The result:** a happier, longer, more active life. To help your heart keep pumping smoothly, and your arteries stay open:

- If you smoke, try your best to quit.

- Keep active with regular exercise.

- Lose extra pounds.

- Avoid fat, especially animal fats, which make your body produce more cholesterol.

- Follow your doctor's advice on when to have your cholesterol level checked.

- Get your blood pressure measured at least once a year and work with your doctor to lower your pressure if it's high.

- At your next visit, ask your doctor about regular doses of aspirin, which studies have shown can significantly lower your risk of heart attack.

That's what is called a heart attack. Without prompt treatment, the damage can progress, permanently weakening the heart — even causing death.

## Are You Having a Heart Attack?

When the heart is under attack, every second counts. Rapid action — including treatment with "clot busting" drugs (tPA or streptokinase) — can stop further damage and restore the heart's regular pumping rhythm. **Chewing and swallowing one aspirin (325 mg) while you seek medical help has been shown to reduce risk of death or complications.**

That's why it's so vital that you learn to recognize the early warning signs of a heart attack.

**Warning Signs.** Most heart attacks involve pain in the center of the chest for at least two minutes. Sometimes the pain travels down the back or arms, particularly the left arm. Or it can spread up the shoulders to the neck, and even to the jaw. Dizziness, fainting, sweating, nausea, shortness of breath or an irregular heartbeat (palpitations) often accompany a heart attack.

During a heart attack, some people experience sustained feelings of squeezing, heaviness or constant pressure in the chest — instead of pain. In contrast, brief, sharp chest pain is almost never a sign of a heart attack.

## Get Help Fast.

*call 911*

If you — or a relative, co-worker or friend — have any of these symptoms, call for emergency help <u>right away</u>. Telephone your local emergency medical system. (Do CPR — cardiopulmonary resuscitation — if the heart attack victim's breathing or pulse stops while waiting for the emergency vehicle.) If you think it would be quicker, drive the victim to the nearest hospital that has round-the-clock emergency cardiac care and clot busters available. Do **not** drive yourself if you think you may be having a heart attack.

**One final tip:** Not all hospitals are equipped to deal with heart attacks. Find out before a crisis which hospitals in your area have 24-hour emergency cardiac care and clot busters available. Then you'll be ready.

"As the arteries grow hard, the heart grows soft." — H.L. Mencken

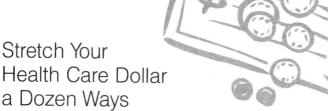

## Stretch Your Health Care Dollar a Dozen Ways

Health care costs just won't stop going up. But if you think there's nothing you can do about it, think again. Here are some personal strategies to help you save on health care and benefit your health in the process:

**1** If you don't already have a family doctor, get one.

By building a relationship with a primary care doctor, you'll get consistent care year after year from a physician who will get to know you and your individual needs well.

**2** Listen carefully to your doctor. But ask
questions, too.

Whenever your doctor suggests a test or treatment — especially
surgery — ask why it's needed, what other options you may have,
and what costs are involved.

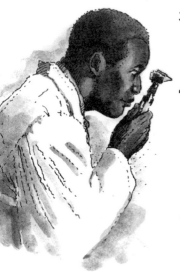

**3** Check all hospital and doctor
bills for errors.

Ask about any items you don't understand.

**4** For minor problems,
call your doctor's office
first to seek self-care advice.

It may save you a visit because many
common symptoms can be handled over
the phone.

**5** Ask your doctor which screening
tests you should have this year.

Mark them in your calendar, and be sure
to show up!

**6** Take advantage of free and low-cost
screening tests...

... such as blood pressure and cholesterol testing at the local mall
or drugstore.

**7** Practice preventive medicine.

Perform your own monthly self-exams: for breast cancer (women),
for testicular cancer (men), and for skin cancer (everyone).

**8** Keep records of when and where you had
X-rays and other tests.

Often, this can save you the expense, hassle and possible pain of
having the same tests repeated all over again unnecessarily.

**9** Reserve emergency rooms for real emergencies.

For chronic health problems, minor illness or injury, the emergency room is actually quite ineffective — and super-expensive.

**10** If you're about to have an operation...

... ask whether it can be done as "day" or "ambulatory" surgery, which is much less costly than staying in a hospital overnight.

**11** Avoid being admitted to a hospital on a weekend.

Most tests and procedures won't be performed until Monday anyway.

**12** Avoid scheduling a hospital stay in July...

... (if at all possible and, of course, if it's not an emergency). July is the start of the medical year, when the doctors-in-training (interns and residents) are just starting out. Studies have shown that patients stay in the hospital longest, and rack up the highest bills ... in July.

"Never go to a doctor whose office plants have died." — Erma Bombeck

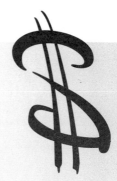

### Money-Saving Medicine

When your doctor writes you a prescription, ask whether you can have any <u>free samples</u> of the medicine being prescribed. Doctors sometimes receive loads of such samples from drug companies and are usually glad to unload them. **Plus:** You save a trip to the pharmacy.

# March

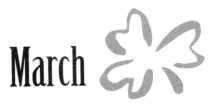

Just when those New Year's resolutions are fading, it's National Nutrition Month — just in time to re-focus on eating right. March is also national Diabetes Alert Month and Workplace Eye Health and Safety Month.

## 6 Simple Tips for a Healthy Diet

### Take one step at a time.

Start eating more whole grains one month, cutting down on butter the following month, reducing the portions of meat the next. (Remember, an official serving of meat is only about 3 ounces, roughly the size of a pack of playing cards.) Gradually, you'll transform your diet!

### Follow a battle plan for grocery shopping.

Shop along the outer aisles of the supermarket first: That's where you'll usually find the healthier items, like fresh fruits, vegetables, bread, fish and low-fat dairy products. Then tackle the center aisles for rice, pasta, dried beans and other basics.

### Buy fewer processed foods.

Why? They're loaded with artificial flavoring, dyes, preservatives, salt and sugar.

### Assert yourself in restaurants.

Order menu items the way you want them. **Examples:** broiled fish instead of fried, and pizza with half the cheese instead of double cheese.

## Cook at home more.

It's the most effective way to make sure your food is healthiest. Weekend cooking can be fun for the whole family, and you can freeze the leftovers to take for lunch.

## Add health boosters to your diet.

You already know about eating less fat, cholesterol and salt. So now go a step further by adding lots of health-enhancing garlic, potassium-rich tropical fruits and cancer-fighting broccoli.

"More die in the United States of too much food than too little." — John Kenneth Galbraith

# Are You at Risk for Diabetes?

**What it is.** When you have diabetes, your body is unable to convert sugar from food into energy. Left untreated, it can lead to kidney failure, gangrene, amputation, blindness, nerve and blood vessel damage, heart disease and stroke. In **Type I**, insulin-dependent diabetes, the body does not produce any insulin, a hormone needed to use food for energy. People with Type I diabetes require daily injections of insulin just to stay alive. In **Type II**, insulin-independent diabetes, the body is unable to make enough insulin or use it properly.

**Who gets it.** Type I diabetes usually strikes children and young adults. But 90 percent of cases are Type II, which occurs most often in people who are over 40 and overweight.

**Who's at risk.** Diabetes tends to run in families. People at greater risk include those with a family history of diabetes, anyone who is overweight or does not exercise regularly and women who have had a baby weighing more than nine pounds. **Also:** Diabetes is more common among African Americans, Hispanics and Native Americans.

**The warning signs.** Type I diabetes often appears suddenly. **Signs and symptoms include:** frequent urination; extreme hunger, thirst or weight loss; weakness; fatigue; moodiness; nausea and high sugar levels in the blood or urine. Type II diabetes often develops slowly and has similar signs and symptoms, plus frequent infections, blurred vision, slow-healing cuts and bruises and tingling or numbness in the hands or feet.

If you're in one of the risk groups mentioned or are concerned, ask your doctor about getting screened for diabetes. With proper treatment and healthy habits, people with diabetes can lead normal, happy lives.

"Above all, do not lose your desire to walk." — Sören Kierkegaard

# Protect Your Vision … for Life

According to one estimate, more than 1,000 eye accidents occur every day. Here's how to prevent one from happening to you … and guard your vision your whole life:

WEAR eye protection such as goggles or shields if your job requires it. Follow all workplace rules and guidelines regarding eye safety; make sure you wear the right kind of eye gear.

USE safeguards at home, where you may be exposed to hot kitchen grease, household cleaners or garden chemicals. Fact is, household products cause more than 32,000 serious eye injuries each year. **Suggestion:** Use a splatter shield in the kitchen and goggles outdoors.

TAKE care when fastening or removing bungee cords. They can easily snap and cause eye injury. Actual injuries reported include: internal bleeding of the eye, dislocated lenses, retinal detachments and even temporary loss of sight.

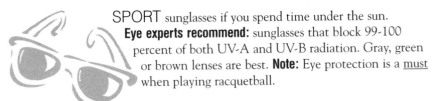

SPORT sunglasses if you spend time under the sun. **Eye experts recommend:** sunglasses that block 99-100 percent of both UV-A and UV-B radiation. Gray, green or brown lenses are best. **Note:** Eye protection is a <u>must</u> when playing racquetball.

EAT right. The vitamins and minerals found in a healthy diet may reduce the risk of eye disorders like cataracts. **Especially helpful:** leafy green vegetables, corn, kiwi, and many other green, red or yellow fruits and vegetables.

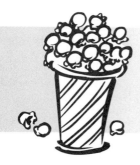

## Eye-Popping News

Popcorn may be good for the eyes. Like all yellow corn, it's rich in lutein and zeaxanthin, carotenoids (pigments) that may help keep your eyes healthy.

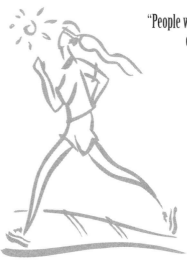

"People who cannot find time for recreation are obliged sooner or later to find time for illness." — John Wanamaker

# April

Serious and not-so-serious, April is National Cancer Control Month, National Alcohol Awareness Month, and a great time to start getting into shape.

## Cancer Prevention: 10 Steps to Take Now

Current research shows many cancers can be prevented by following some simple dos and don'ts. Your cancer fighting strategy must include not only building up natural defenses with a smart diet and lifestyle, but also cutting down on anything that may increase your chances of getting this disease. It could save your life.

## 1 Eat plenty of fiber-rich foods.

You'll find fiber abundant in fruits, vegetables, whole grains and legumes (dried beans). Although one recent study suggested that fiber does not lower the risk of colorectal (large bowel) cancer, on the whole, research still shows that fiber lowers your risk. Overall, the more fiber, the bulkier the stools, and the more fruits and vegetables, the lower the risk of colon cancer.

## 2 Choose foods packed with vitamins A, C and beta carotene.

**Best choices:** carrots, peaches, grapefruit, oranges, squash, tomatoes, sweet peppers and sweet potatoes. Don't rely on high doses of vitamin supplements because too much of a good thing could be harmful!

## 3 Discover the cabbage family.

Broccoli, cauliflower, Brussels sprouts and kale may protect against cancers of the lung, stomach and colon.

## 4 Drink tea.

Especially helpful may be the green types, such as chamomile tea, which contain substances called polyphenols. These substances are antioxidants and may help protect against a variety of cancers.

## 5 Control your weight.

Obesity is linked to cancers of the gallbladder, colon, breast and uterus.

## 6 Exercise regularly.

Research suggests it may help protect against the development of colorectal, breast and prostate cancers.

## 7 Don't smoke, chew or sniff tobacco.

These habits are responsible for one-third of all cancer deaths and have been linked not only to lung cancer but also to cancers of the mouth and throat — and possibly even of the bladder, pancreas, kidney and white blood cells.

## 8 Trim fat off your diet.

Eating less fat, especially animal fat from meat and dairy products, is believed to help decrease your risk of cancers of the colon and prostate.

## 9 If you drink, do so in moderation.

Heavy alcohol use may raise the risk of several cancers, including breast, mouth and throat cancers.

## 10 Protect yourself from the sun.

Avoid overexposure, and use sunscreen when out in direct sunlight — look for SPF 15 or higher on the sunscreen's label.

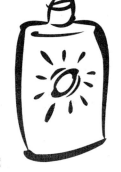

*"It is not the years in your life but the life in your years that counts." — Adlai Stevenson*

## None for the Road

Each year, alcohol-related accidents result in approximately 17,500 deaths in the United States. In addition, impaired driving is a leading cause of death among people 25 years and under. Don't be a statistic; keep these simple rules in mind:

## Be a responsible host.

- If serving alcohol, have high-protein foods such as cheese, meats and shrimp available.

- Have non-alcoholic drinks and non-carbonated mixers on hand (carbonated beverages make the body absorb alcohol faster).

- Stop serving alcohol about 2 hours before the party is over, and serve dessert and coffee instead.

- Don't let guests drive after drinking alcohol. Call a taxi or a friend.

- <u>Never</u> serve alcohol to someone under 21.

- Be a responsible driver. Don't drink alcohol and drive. Arrange for transportation if you plan on drinking.

- <u>Never</u> ride in a car with someone who has been drinking.

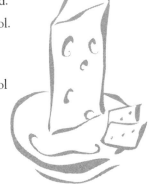

## Alcohol facts:

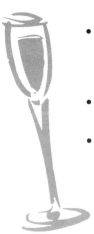

- Alcohol slows your reactions. Alcohol makes you less alert but may give you a false sense of confidence.

- Alcohol affects your judgment. You will not be able to judge speeds and distances. Alcohol also affects your judgment of how fit you are to drive — you may believe you're driving better than you actually are.

- Time is the only thing that can sober you — not coffee or a cold shower.

- Just one drink can affect you — even if your blood alcohol level is below the legal limit.

# Spring
# Slim-Down

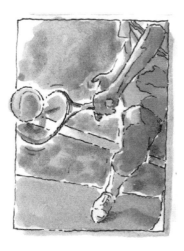

Like death and taxes, weight is governed by laws you can't escape. And being overweight raises the risk of a variety of health problems, including diabetes, heart disease — and even arthritis and back pain.

But you don't have to become overweight — or stay that way. The main equation is simple:

**The food you eat - the energy you spend = your extra weight**

How to slim down? Exercise more and eat less. It's best to eat smaller portions of a healthy diet while stepping up your exercise routine. **The reason:** Working out helps reverse the slowdown in the body's metabolic "burn rate" that can result from eating less. If you can tinker with only one element, opt for exercise, not diet. Just by exercising more, while eating the same, you can lose body fat, inches and sizes — even if you don't lose pounds. Studies suggest weight lost through exercise alone may be easier to keep off.

Keeping It Off. Losing weight is relatively easy. What's hard is keeping it off. Dieters often resort to their old habits (overeating and inactivity), gaining back their weight — and then some. The regained weight tends to be higher in fat and lower in muscle. So if you let your weight yo-yo, you just get flabbier.

How to achieve lifelong weight control? Exercise regularly, and eat controlled portions of a variety of foods. Don't entirely eliminate all your favorite foods or you might start craving them. Instead, learn to enjoy them sparingly. By eating less fatty foods, you'll consume fewer total calories. You can substitute foods rich in fiber, which makes you feel full. Some recent studies indicate a low-fat diet is more slimming than a fatty one, even with the same number of total calories.

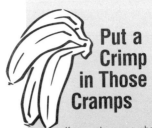

## Put a Crimp in Those Cramps

If you get cramps when you work out, try drinking more water, since dehydration may be a factor. A mineral imbalance may be another culprit; try adding more potassium to your diet. **Good sources:** baked potatoes … bananas … cantaloupes. **Tip:** Taking extra calcium may also help.

"Laughter is internal jogging."
— Norman Cousins

Don't weigh yourself more than once a week, so you won't feel discouraged — or elated — about fleeting "water weight" ups and downs. **And remember:** A slow, steady weight loss — no more than one or two pounds a week — is easiest to maintain. The turtle beats the hare at the slimming race.

**Exercise Rx.** Walk, bike, swim, skate, dance or run. If you're out of shape, start small — for instance, with a one-mile walk. Gradually build up to three 20-minute workouts a week. During each workout, your heart should beat faster than usual, but without your getting breathless.

**How Big a Portion?** Standard portion sizes are much smaller than you probably think. **The main example:** A portion of meat is <u>only 3 ounces</u>. So a one-pound steak is more than five dinners' worth. If standard portions seem too little, try serving them on smaller plates — chew your food slowly and savor it.

# May

A merry, merry month, indeed.
Warmer weather means more opportunities to get up out of that easy chair (it's National Bike Month). You'll be happier if you control any allergies you may have (it's Asthmas and Allergy Awareness Month), and sleep easier (Better Sleep Month) knowing your blood pressure is under control (it's National High Blood Pressure Month, too).

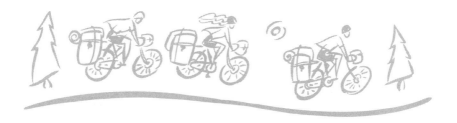

# Cycling Fun & Fitness

Looking for an especially fun way to get in shape? One you'll really stick with? One you can do alone or with friends? In town or out in the woods? **Consider cycling.**

Outdoors on a bike, cycling can transform your workout into an adventure. One-speed or 21-speed, fancy or plain, a bike is your ticket to explore your neighborhood and discover new places. And in the process you'll enjoy a wealth of health benefits.

Like other aerobic exercises — such as brisk walking, jogging, swimming, skating and jumping rope — cycling involves sustained, repetitive action of large muscle groups. Regular aerobic activity can help you lose extra weight and maintain your ideal weight once you've reached it. Cycling at 12 miles per hour, a 150-pound person burns 410 calories an hour. Regular aerobic exercise, such as cycling, can also help lower your blood pressure, as well as the levels of "bad" (LDL) cholesterol and triglycerides (fat) in your blood. Together, these beneficial effects can <u>cut</u> your heart risk.

"<u>Aerobicizing</u>" is a healthy way to work off stress. You'll probably find it makes you feel more energetic. And it's great for your mind, too — not just your body — helping to stave off depressed feelings. <u>Cycling</u> can be a valuable part of a cross-training program, in which you switch from one activity to another.

## Why cross-train? 
Working the same muscles the same way at every workout can overstress them. But cycling works your leg muscles differently than does walking or jogging. Try starting with one 30-minute bike ride, every other day. Especially if your muscles are sore the next day, take a day off cycling.

"Youth is not a time of life — it is a state of mind." — Anonymous

# Play It Safe

Each year, American cyclists have over a million serious accidents. Most involve kids under 14, so you should teach your children these cycling safety basics — and set a good example by following them yourself.

**Most important:** Wear a helmet. Helmets have been shown to lower the risk of head injury in bike crashes.
**And that risk is real:** Head injuries account for 85 percent of the nation's 1,000 yearly cycling deaths. When you buy a helmet, check for an approval sticker from ANSI (the American National Standards Institute). New models weigh less than a pound, so they're plenty comfortable. **Also:**

- Follow the rules of the road, obeying the same traffic laws and signals as cars.
- Equip your bike with lights and reflectors that are clearly visible to motorists, in case you ever have to do any risky night riding.
- Stay in the bike lane, if there is one, don't dart in and out of traffic, and keep your distance from parked cars — you never know when a car door might open.
- Don't use a personal stereo when cycling outside, as this distracts you and blocks out warning sounds from other traffic.

# Surprising Facts About Blood Pressure... and What You Can Do About It

Concerned about blood pressure? Here's what you need to know. Blood pressure is tracked with two numbers: The higher number (called systolic) is the pressure when your heart contracts; the lower one (diastolic), when it relaxes. If it's elevated (135/85 or higher), you need to work with your doctor to get it under control.

**1**    The cause of high blood pressure isn't known in nine of 10 cases. But the disorder is easy to detect and usually simple to control.

**2**    Nearly 64 million Americans age 6 and older have high blood pressure — including 1.5 million kids age 6 to 9.

**3**   Of those people who have high blood pressure, nearly a third have no idea that they have it. **The reason:** It causes no pain or symptoms.

**4**   Generally, the older you get, the <u>higher</u> your blood pressure.

**5**   Women age 65 and older are more likely to have high blood pressure than men.

**6**   High blood pressure tends to run in families.

**7**   People of African, Latino or Hispanic roots are more likely to have high blood pressure than white Americans.

**8**   High blood pressure strains the heart by making it work harder to pump enough blood and oxygen to the body's organs.

**9**   When the heart works harder than normal for a long time, it tends to enlarge, and an enlarged heart can fail to meet its demands.

**10**   High blood pressure contributes to hardening of the arteries, heart attacks, strokes, blindness and kidney failure.

**11**   Getting high blood pressure treated can stop — and even repair — kidney damage caused by the disorder.

**12**   Anger can raise blood pressure.

**13**   Regularly drinking too much alcohol can raise blood pressure in some people.

**14**   Smoking cigarettes can make high blood pressure harder to control.

**15**   Eating too much licorice candy can raise blood pressure (<u>real</u> licorice, not the common, artificially flavored kind).

**16**   One in four people with high blood pressure could get the condition under control simply by switching to a healthier way of life — without any medication.

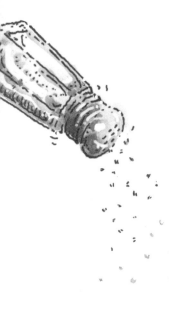

## Hypertension Self-Defense

- Get your blood pressure tested at least once a year.
- Lose extra weight.
- Exercise regularly.
- Cut down on salt.
- Eat more fresh fruits and low-fat dairy products, for pressure-lowering potassium and calcium.
- Channel your anger, and cope with stress.
- If your doctor prescribes a pressure-lowering medication, be sure to take it regularly and on time.

"The trouble with life in the fast lane is that you get to the other end in an awful hurry." — John Jensen

## Hay Fever Self-Defense

About 35 million Americans are allergic to tree and grass pollen and are subject to "seasonal allergic rhinitis," otherwise known as hay fever. **The good news:** Trying these strategies can help minimize the misery ...

1   Reduce exposure. Try to schedule outdoor activities when the pollen count is low and at daybreak when plants are still covered with dew ... at night ... after a steady rain ... on cloudy, humid, windless days. **Surprising:** Thunderstorms don't help because large raindrops are inefficient at washing pollen from the air.

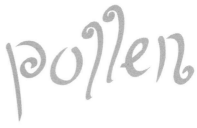

# pollen

**2** Enjoy the indoors. Indoor air is relatively free of pollen, so keep windows closed when you can. Allergists recommend air-conditioning in cars and homes for ventilation and cooling. **More help:** Extra-sensitive sufferers may benefit from using an air-cleaning machine with a high-efficiency particle air filter.

**3** Avoid common irritants. Try to steer clear of tobacco smoke, automobile exhaust, laundry detergents, insecticide sprays, hair spray and perfume. **Useful:** Wash your hands <u>frequently</u> and keep them away from the eyes ... wash hair at night to remove any pollen and keep it from settling on pillows and bedding.

**4** Control symptoms. Over-the-counter antihistamines, which help block allergic reactions, are most effective if taken before symptoms surface. **Trap:** The drowsiness they can produce. **Solution:** Avoid these drugs whenever safety requires you to stay alert, or speak to your doctor about prescription antihistamines that work without the drowsiness.

"Always be a little kinder than necessary." — James M. Barrie
(Peter Pan author)

## Car Talk

Up to a third of all auto air conditioners are infected with fungi, a problem for allergy and asthma sufferers. **Actions:** Keep car windows partly open for 10-15 minutes after turning on the air conditioner ... use fresh air rather than recirculated air ... have your car treated with special disinfectant, available at auto dealers, some service stations and most auto air conditioner shops.

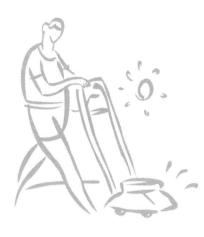

# June

Summer's here: time to work on the house and the yard, time to step up your exercise routine (if you haven't already), and time to kick back and relax. It's also National Safety Month and National Men's Health Week (June 11-17).

## 4 Steps that Protect Your Knees

Itching to get out and run? Before you do, here's some staggering news: An estimated 50 million Americans suffer from knee problems. It's easy to understand why. Running, dancing or even house cleaning, your knees undergo a lot of stress. Fact is, simply climbing stairs can put pressure on each knee equal to **four times** your body weight. **To minimize the impact:**

CHECK your feet. Flat feet, feet that roll inward too much when you walk or poor leg alignment can put greater stress on your knee joints. **Action:** Keep your knee in line with your foot when walking, running or biking. **Self-defense:** A custom-made arch support can help correct many foot or alignment problems.

INSPECT your shoes. **Beware:** If shoes are very worn or ill-fitting, they may put your knees at risk.

STRETCH. **Why:** Tight leg muscles result in extra strain on the knees. **Good start:** Stretch legs regularly, especially <u>before and after</u> exercise.

STRENGTHEN. **For stronger knees:** Sit on a desk or counter and hold onto the edge. Slowly raise one leg, extending the knee completely. Hold for five seconds, and then lower slowly. Repeat ten times, and then switch legs. **Even better:** Add ankle weights if desired.

**ALREADY HAVE KNEE PROBLEMS?** Avoid activities that cause you to put weight on your bent knees, like climbing hills and stairs, kneeling, squatting, and hard-on-the-knee sports such as football, soccer, squash, tennis, skiing and running on concrete.

# A Fly in the Ointment

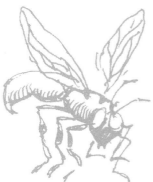

DEET, the active ingredient in most insect repellants, can lower the effectiveness of sunscreens by about 30 percent. So take extra caution against the sun when using both.

# 5 Deadly Combinations

## Ladders and Wires.

Since aluminum conducts electricity, ladders made of this material can be hazardous if used near electrical wires. Besides, aluminum ladders are so lightweight that sudden movements or strong winds can sometimes knock them over. **For your safety:** Use a wooden or fiberglass ladder, not an aluminum one, when working on your house.

## Bleach and Ammonia.

When chlorine bleach is combined with ammonia cleaners or with ammonia-containing dishwashing liquids (like Dawn, Joy, Ivory or Palmolive), it can give off a poisonous gas that can instantly inflame your lungs. **For your safety:** <u>Always</u> read labels first, before mixing any chemicals.

## Medications and Medicines.

All medications — prescription and over-the-counter — can cause side effects and interfere with each other. **For your safety:** Whenever starting any new medication, remind your doctor or pharmacist of any drugs you are currently taking.

## Smoking and Driving.

Smokers can get distracted while handling cigarettes, lighters and ashtrays. They have one-and-a-half times more car accidents than nonsmokers. **For your safety:** Not just "Don't drink and drive," but also "Don't smoke and drive."

## Storms and Utilities.

Plumbing and phone equipment can conduct electricity if lightning strikes your building. **For your safety:** During thunderstorms, avoid bathing, showering and using regular and cellular telephones.

**"If you want the rainbow, you gotta put up with the rain." — Dolly Parton**

# Great Ways to Guard Dad's Health

**Reminder:** Father's Day is Sunday, June 17. Whether the "Dad" you'll be honoring is your father, a grandfather, uncle, husband, brother or co-worker, let him know you want him around for many years by:

**1** Giving him "gifts of good health."
Ask your local hospital if it offers gift certificates for cholesterol and blood pressure screenings or nutrition counseling. If you give Dad one of these, offer to go with him to make sure he redeems it.

**2** Arranging a weekly walk-and-talk.
If Dad lives nearby, set aside a special time for a brisk half-hour walk together. You'll both be doing your cardiovascular systems a favor, to say nothing of the psychological and emotional benefits of "connecting." If Dad lives far away, help him find a walking buddy.

**3** Making sure he gets the checkups he needs.

Regular physical exams include screenings that help Dad catch little problems before they become big ones. The critical checklist includes tests for colorectal and prostate cancer, blood pressure monitoring, and vaccines for flu and pneumonia. Have Dad contact his health care provider between now and next Father's Day to establish a game plan if he doesn't already have one.

**4** Getting him to the eye doctor.

It's wise for everyone to consider regular vision checkups. If Dad is diabetic or African American, or if there's a family history of glaucoma, he should also inquire about screening for this leading cause of blindness.

### Men: Burn to Beat Cancer

In a recent study from the Harvard School of Public Health, men who burned 3,000 calories or more a week while working out were 39 percent less likely to develop lung cancer than less active men. That's about 6-8 hours of moderate exercise every week.

**The bottom line:**
Take these steps, and you get the best gift of all — a happier, healthier "Dad."

# July

It's hot. The neighbors are on vacation. Folks at work are finding reasons to duck out early on Fridays. And you're planning your own good times: days at the beach, fireworks on the 4th, tooling in the garden. This month, some thoughts on how to guard your health through it all.

# The Miracle Drink

Next time you raise a glass to good health, fill it with water. Water helps every living cell in your body; in fact, your body is really about two-thirds water. And, did you know that you can survive up to 30 days without food ... but only 72 hours without water?

Day to day, poor hydration can make you feel "not quite right." Losing just 5-10 percent of your fluids — that's 2-5 quarts — can lead to mild dizziness, headache, lethargy and difficulty thinking. Right off the bat you lose about 10 cups of water each day through sweat, exhaled air and waste. But it's especially important to maintain your fluids during the summer, when you can lose up to a quart an hour. As with a car, keeping the proper water level can prevent a breakdown.

**Some simple dos and don'ts: Do** drink a glass of pure water about 20 minutes before heavy physical activity, and **do** drink half a glass every 15 minutes during activity. **Don't** rely on caffeinated and alcoholic beverages for fluid. They'll make you urinate more and raise your fluid needs. **Don't** trust your thirst completely — experts say your body shuts off its "thirsty" signal before you've drunk enough. **Recommendation:** Drink at least two or three tall glasses of water daily beyond what your thirst tells you to.

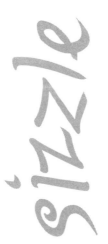

# "The Good, the Bad and the Ugly"

The sun is hot stuff. With a surface temperature of about 10,000° F, its starring role is to supply all of the energy supporting life on earth. But beware: This leading player can be both hero and villain ...

**The Good.** Sunshine can prompt the brain to release chemicals that help you feel energized. In fact, one study showed that sun exposure actually helped improve work productivity. And the sun's rays help your body manufacture vitamin D, which promotes bone-building by aiding in the body's absorption of calcium and phosphorous.

**The Bad.** Sun exposure can raise your risk of eye problems like cataracts (clouding of the lens inside the eye). And it's estimated that 9 out of 10 skin cancers could have been prevented by protection from the sun's rays.

**Recommended:** Select sunglasses whose labels say they block 99-100 percent of both UV-A and UV-B radiation. Gray, green or brown lenses are best. Limit sun exposure between 10 AM and 3 PM, apply waterproof sunscreen 15-30 minutes before going outside, and wear a wide-brim hat and tight-weave clothing.

**The Ugly.** Sun-induced premature skin aging often results in wrinkled, loose, leathery skin that's densely freckled, dry and dotted with brown splotches called age or liver spots. Eventually, spidery red lines may develop, as may precancerous blemishes called actinic keratoses. These usually look like small, scaly light pink or reddish patches and need to be seen by a skin doctor. But the good news is that your skin has a remarkable ability to repair itself and can even partly reverse the effects of this "photoaging" — if you protect it from further sun exposure. So rub in the sunscreen ... cover up ... and keep looking young.

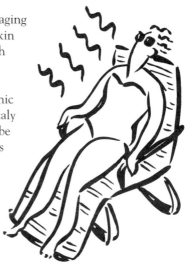

# Take the 30-Second Hearing Test

While it's true that sudden loud noises, such as 4th of July fireworks, can temporarily damage your hearing, the main cause of permanent hearing loss is the day to day pounding your ears are subjected to from our noisy society.

 **Try this:** In a quiet room, keep this book at arm's length on a flat surface and scratch the spot to the left with your fingernail. Or sit down, cross your feet and rub your shoes together. Either sound is equivalent to a whisper. If you have difficulty hearing them, it's a good idea to have your hearing checked.

# How to Outsmart Poison Ivy

The real culprit behind the rash, blisters and itch caused by poison ivy is urushiol (uh-ROO-she-all), an allergy-producing chemical in the sap of poison ivy and its cousins, poison oak and sumac. It can remain active on contaminated objects for months or even years.

About 85 percent of people are sensitive to urushiol, although it may take several exposures to trigger an allergic reaction. **Here's how to avoid the itch:**

- Know the enemy. Poison ivy leaves usually cluster in threes. They may be dull but tend to be shiny, with smooth or saw-toothed edges. Blossoms appear in late spring, white berries in late summer.

- Cover up. If you're in an area where these plants grow, wear gloves and other protective clothing. Avoid lightweight fabrics, since urushiol can penetrate them.

- Use extra caution. Urushiol can be transferred from any contaminated object, including pets' fur, clothing, firewood, hands — even a gardening tool you haven't used in a year. So avoid the ivy, but also try not to touch anything you think has been exposed, including pets.

- Act fast. Urushiol can penetrate the skin in minutes. So rinse exposed areas with cold running water right away and scrub under fingernails. Wash clothing and other objects with strong detergent, and wipe off shoes.

**For relief:** For mild cases, cold compresses, cool baths, calamine lotion or over-the-counter hydrocortisone products can help. But if you've had severe reactions in the past, it's best to consult a dermatologist without delay after a new exposure.

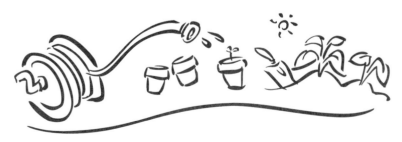

# What to Do
# for Sun Blisters

Sun or heat-burn blisters are best left alone. Medical studies show that if ruptured, peeled or needled they are more likely to get infected.

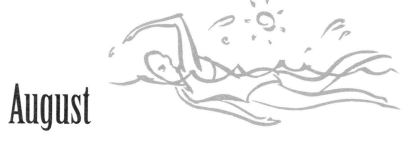

# August

During these dog days of summer, remember that summer is a season that carries its own safety risks. The more active you are, the more you need to take precautions against potential hazards.

## Avoid These Summer Bummers

Every year, the great outdoors is a little less great for people who encounter other, potentially dangerous "outdoor types." To play it safe, watch out for these problems:

WATER BUGS. Even water that looks clean may contain tiny, disease-causing organisms, bacteria or parasites. So when hiking, resist the temptation to drink from a cool, running brook. **For safety:** Bring your own water supply. If you can't, use purification tablets or boil the water for 10 minutes first.

INSECT STINGS. For those who are highly sensitive, a single sting from a bee, wasp or hornet can cause death if left untreated. So if you have a known allergy to insect stings, keep a bee-sting kit with you at all times. And seek medical attention <u>immediately</u> if a severe allergic reaction develops (usually within half an hour): shortness of breath, wheezing, swelling of the face or fainting.

**TICK TROUBLE.** Ticks can transmit illnesses like Lyme disease. **Self-defense:** In wooded areas or fields with tall grass, wear long pants tucked into your socks, a long-sleeve shirt and hat. Choose light-colored clothing, which makes ticks easier to spot. Apply a repellent containing permethrin to clothing and let it dry before dressing; use an insect repellent containing DEET on exposed skin.

**SNAKE BITES. Remember:** A snake can strike up to half its length. So maintain <u>at least</u> six feet between you and any snake you see. Keep hands out of hidden places, such as under rocks or firewood. Stay out of tall grass unless you're wearing thick leather boots ... stick to hiking paths ... and be extra careful when climbing rocks — one of a snake's favorite hiding places.

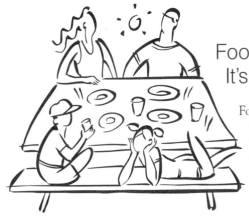

# Food Poisoning:
# It's No Picnic

Food poisoning strikes up to a third of all Americans each year. Warm weather marks the beginning of peak food poisoning season. **Why?** Picnic and barbecue foods aren't always kept cold or hot enough to prevent bacterial growth.

While most people suffer only short-term (1-8 days) vomiting and diarrhea, some food poisonings can result in permanent nerve damage, kidney failure or death. Here are some basic rules to keep your food safe:

## KEEP HOT FOODS HOT AND COLD FOODS COLD

Store foods below 40° F or keep warm above 140° F. Don't keep perishables in the car. Don't eat perishable foods (meats, fish, cooked vegetables, dairy products and eggs) that were left out in temperatures between 40° F and 140° F for more than three hours.

## COOK RAW MEATS, POULTRY, EGGS AND SEAFOODS THOROUGHLY

The general rule is to heat to 160° F. Some heat-resistant spores are not killed during cooking, so store perishables safely below 40° F.

## EXAMINE FOOD BEFORE EATING

Throw out food with off-odors, visible slime, mold or off-color.

## WASH HANDS WELL

Wash hands with soap and hot water. If there's no water available at your picnic site, use antibacterial hand gels available at retail outlets.

## PREVENT CROSS-CONTAMINATION

Wash cutting boards, countertops and other surfaces with soap and water. Rinse with a bleach-water solution if they came in contact with raw meat, fish or poultry. Don't use wooden cutting boards to cut raw foods or meats. **Reason:** Wood is porous and bacteria can grow. Don't combine leftovers with fresh foods.

## BARBECUE BASICS

When barbecuing, don't put cooked foods on the same plate that held the raw food. The same marinade shouldn't be used to baste meat during cooking if it was used to marinate raw meat.

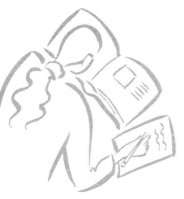

# September

As back-to-school time looms, it's time to get educated ... with National Cholesterol Education Awareness Month, Prostate Cancer Awareness Month and 5-a-Day for Better Health Week (September 9-15).

# Cholesterol: The Facts

Everything you ever wanted to know but were afraid to ask:

1 **What is cholesterol?** It's a soft, waxy substance that helps transport fat through your blood vessels and is used in cell metabolism. Your liver produces almost all the cholesterol your body needs.

2 **Why is it harmful?** Cholesterol containing plaques can build up in arterial walls and cause narrowing of the arteries, slowing or blocking blood flow to vital organs. High total cholesterol (240 mg/dl or greater) is a known risk factor for heart attack. The desirable range is lower than 200, with 200-239 considered "borderline high."

3 **Explain "good" and "bad" cholesterol.** Cholesterol is hauled through the blood-stream by molecules called lipoproteins. Low-density lipoproteins (LDL) tend to deposit cholesterol in arterial walls. High-density lipoproteins (HDL) help sweep cholesterol out of the system. Thus, HDL cholesterol is referred to as "good" and LDL cholesterol as "bad." An HDL of 35 or higher and LDL lower than 130 are desirable.

4 **What's this I hear about "total-to-HDL ratio"?** Some doctors express cholesterol levels as a ratio of total blood cholesterol to HDL. The goal is to keep the ratio below 4.5 to one. **To calculate:** Divide your total cholesterol by your HDL level. **Example:** 200÷50=4, or 4:1.

5 **What about this new risk factor called "homocysteine"?**
Ho-mo-SIS-teen is an amino acid in the blood. Too much may be bad for your heart. **Why:** High levels of homocysteine may cause the arteries to thicken and scar; cholesterol then builds up in the scarred tissues. **To lower:** Eat a varied diet to get vitamins B6, B12 and folic acid. Ideal homocysteine levels are below 9 "micromoles." If levels are very high, B6, B12 and folic acid supplements can often bring them down to desirable range.

**6** How often should I have my cholesterol checked? At least every five years — but more frequently if your total cholesterol is elevated, HDL is low, or you have other risk factors for coronary artery disease. Check with your doctor.

**To raise HDL and lower LDL:** Try aerobic exercise ... drink only in moderation ... don't smoke ... lose excess weight ... eat fewer saturated and "trans" fats and use more olive oil.

## The Napkin Test

How to tell if a cracker is too fatty to eat? Rub a paper napkin on it. If the cracker leaves a grease mark, it has too much oil. Even though vegetable oil is healthier than animal fat, it's still high in calories and best eaten in moderation.

# Eating Right — Veggies That Boost Your Health

What do veggies have going for them? They're naturally cholesterol-free, low in calories and (except for avocados) virtually free of fat. Vegetables — especially unpeeled, with their skins on — are high in fiber. They're full of needed vitamins and minerals. And they offer a delicious array of different flavors: from the tangy taste of collard greens to the sweetness of a fresh carrot.

### The Orange and the Green. Orange and green vegetables have special benefits. For instance, orange (and yellow and red) vegetables — especially carrots — are rich in beta-carotene, which some researchers believe may protect against cancer. Also, the body converts beta-carotene to vitamin A, which is needed for good vision, particularly in the dark. And green leafy vegetables are good sources of iron, calcium and a B vitamin called folic acid.

Ideally you should eat at least one serving of a green leafy vegetable and one of the orange type every day. And in choosing your produce, the darker the green and the brighter the orange, red or yellow, the better. Here are some health choices:

**Orange, Yellow and Red Vegetables:** Carrots, sweet potatoes, tomatoes, red peppers, pumpkin and yellow and orange squash

**Green Leafy Vegetables:** Spinach, lettuce, kale, collard greens, mustard greens, broccoli, asparagus — and try "gourmet" greens (like arugula, chicory, escarole, Swiss chard and dandelion greens)

**Remember:** You should try to get 5-9 servings of veggies and fruit every day. **Ideas:** Add fruit to cereal at breakfast … snack on raw vegetables instead of potato chips … visit the salad bar at lunch … sip juice instead of coffee, tea or soda.

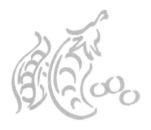

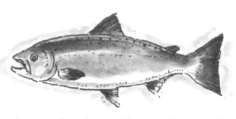

## Prostate Cancer Self-Defense

Cancer of the prostate — the walnut-sized male gland located between the bladder and the rectum — is the second leading cause of cancer death in men. The good news is that it can often be treated successfully when found early. So know the facts:

PREVENTION. The exact cause of prostate cancer isn't known, so doctors can't say for certain how to prevent it. However, studies have linked prostate cancer with eating saturated fat. A report in the *Journal of the National Cancer Institute* found that those less likely to die from prostate cancer favored soy foods, fish, cereals and nuts over foods high in saturated fats. So replacing animal fats and red meat with plant foods and fish seems a sensible "can't hurt, could help" strategy.

**DETECTION.** The best ways doctors have to spot prostate cancer early remain the PSA test — a simple blood test to detect levels of prostate-specific antigen — and a digital rectal exam (DRE). The American Cancer Society recommends that all men over 50 talk to their doctors about having both tests. Men in high-risk groups (African Americans and men with close family members who have had prostate cancer) should ask about screening sooner.

**IMMEDIATE ACTION.** Consult a physician if you notice <u>any</u> of these warning signs: difficulty urinating, blood in the urine, pain in the pelvic or low back area lasting several weeks or more, loss of appetite and weight, noticeably frequent or urgent urination or frequent urination at night. **Note:** Although urination problems may be a sign of prostate cancer, more often they're a sign of a less serious disease known as benign prostate hyperplasia.

## You'll Say Tomato

A recent review of 72 studies in the *Journal of the National Cancer Institute* found that people who ate the most tomatoes and tomato-based products had a consistently lower risk of cancer — especially prostate, lung and stomach cancers. **Note:** Some research indicates that foods with cooked tomatoes — such as tomato sauce — are best.

# October

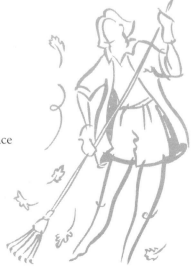

October is loaded with official health observances, perhaps because health organizations believe it's their last chance to get the nation's attention before the holidays gear up. Among the many worthy observances are National Spinal Health Month, National Breast Cancer Awareness Month, and National Crime Prevention Month.

# Best Ways You Can Beat Back Pain — Fast!

Four out of five adults suffer back pain at some point in their lives. Fortunately, it goes away 90 percent of the time. Here's what you can do when lower back pain strikes:

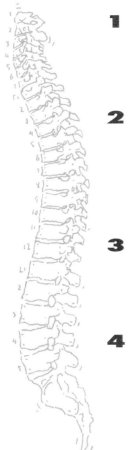

**1** Apply relief. A heating pad or ice pack — whichever feels best — may ease much of your discomfort. If needed, take a non-prescription pain reliever containing ibuprofen, aspirin, naproxen, ketoprofen or acetaminophen.

**2** Go to bed. If your pain is severe, consider 1-2 days of complete bed rest, getting up for meals or to go to the bathroom. **But remember:** Too much bed rest can actually be <u>bad</u> for your back. Experts say longer than 48 hours may weaken the muscles that help support the spine and delay your recovery.

**3** Get in the right position. When lying down, use a firm, comfortable mattress and avoid sleeping on your stomach. Instead, lie either on your side with your knees bent or on your back with a pillow tucked under your knees.

**4** Try carrying on as usual. Recent studies suggest that continuing normal activities as pain allows may speed recovery even better than bed rest or back exercises. But do remember to limit lifting, twisting, bending, prolonged sitting or wearing high heels — all of which can further strain your spine.

When to Get Help. While most back pain isn't caused by anything serious, it sometimes results from damage to the disks that cushion the bones of the spine. This may require further treatment. Call your doctor if symptoms persist for more than 3-4 weeks, or if pain greatly limits activities, steadily worsens or travels down the leg.

Other symptoms could mean more serious conditions like bone fracture or even cancer. Signs to seek immediate medical attention include: tingling or weakness in arms or legs, pain accompanied by fever, bowel or bladder problems, numbness in the groin or rectal area or if you've had cancer.

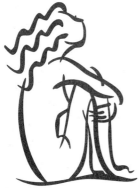

# The Good News About Breast Cancer

Many women are alarmed by the fast-rising statistics about their likelihood of developing breast cancer. The risks are serious. But there's plenty a woman can do to keep the threat in perspective and under control.

One explanation for the rise in breast cancer cases is improved screening, which detects more tumors, and sooner than before. That's good news, because effective screening saves lives by catching cancer at earlier stages, when it responds best to treatment. In fact, prompt detection is the most powerful strategy in the fight against breast cancer.

Who's At Risk. Unfortunately, breast cancer runs in families. A woman's risk is doubled if her mother, daughter or sister has had the disease — and raised, though less so, if her aunt or grandmother has had it. But remember, as any woman ages her odds of developing breast cancer rise dramatically. So it pays for every woman to make early breast cancer detection a top priority throughout her life.

Self-Defense. Though you can't stop aging, some research suggests that it might help to take the following actions now. And it certainly couldn't hurt.

- If you smoke, quit. (Some studies link smoking to breast cancer, as well as lung cancer.)
- Eat a balanced diet — lower in fat and higher in fiber.
- Exercise regularly and lose any extra weight. (Generally, the larger the breasts, the harder to feel a lump.)
- Curb your use of alcohol and caffeine. (Large quantities may raise breast cancer risks.)

To boost their chance of finding breast cancer early, all women should check their own breasts once a month, starting at age 20. Here's how:

- Set a consistent time: for example, four days after each menstrual period (or the first day of the month).
- Feel each of your breasts thoroughly while standing or sitting — and again while lying down.
- Move your fingers in a slow spiral, starting around each nipple, and work your way outward in widening circles.
- Look at your breasts in a mirror with your arms at your sides, then raised and then with hands pressed against your hips.
- Do see your doctor promptly if you notice a lump or other change in either breast.
- **But don't panic:** Most lumps turn out to be non-cancerous, though they're worth following up.

According to the American Cancer Society, every woman should also get her breasts examined by a doctor or nurse at least once every three years after age 20 — and yearly after age 40. And women should talk to their doctors about having mammograms (special low-dose X-ray pictures of the breasts) taken every one or two years starting at age 40 — and yearly after age 50.

**The bottom line:** There's much a woman can do to detect breast cancer early — and to minimize its impact on her life in case she does develop the disease.

"A pessimist is someone who complains about the noise when opportunity knocks."
— Michael Levine, author

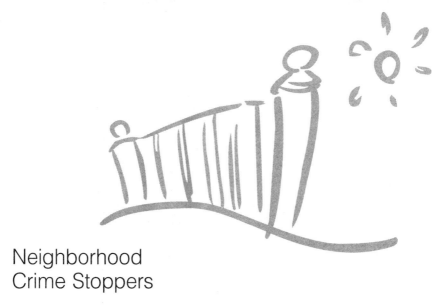

# Neighborhood Crime Stoppers

Your neighborhood should be a welcoming and safe place to relax. Unfortunately, the increase in two-income families also increases the community's vulnerability to crime. That's why it's important for neighbors to keep an eye out for suspicious behavior — anything that seems slightly "out of place."

### Examples of suspicious behavior:

- A stranger entering your neighbor's house when it is unoccupied.

- Anyone removing accessories, license plates or gas from a car.

- Persons loitering around your neighborhood, schools, and parks.

- Anyone forcing entrance to, or tampering with, a residence or vehicle.

- Someone going door-to-door in your neighborhood. Check identification of all solicitors, meter readers, and repairmen prior to allowing entry.

- One or more juveniles walking casually through the neighborhood looking into houses, automobiles, backyards, etc.

- Persons exhibiting unusual mental or physical symptoms.

- Traffic to and from a certain residence on a daily or very regular basis, especially during late or unusual hours.

- Any vehicle moving slowly and without lights or following a course that appears aimless or repetitive, or parked, occupied vehicles.

- Business transactions conducted from a car.

- A flashlight beam in a neighbor's home when they are away.

Call 911 or your local law enforcement when you suspect something. When you call, you should be able to tell them: What happened? When? Where? Give them a description of person(s) and/or vehicle including license number, make, model, color, any noticeable damage and direction of travel.

## Outfox a Burglar

- 73 percent of thieves enter homes through windows, not doors. **Simple safeguard:** Storm windows.

- Many burglars cut phone lines before breaking in. **Simple safeguard:** A notice saying police will automatically be summoned if the phone lines are cut.

- The easy way for a thief to see if you're home is to look in the garage for your car. **Simple safeguard:** Cover all garage windows.

# November

Is it already holiday time again? Statistics show that the average person gains a whopping <u>six pounds</u> between Thanksgiving and New Year's. Not you, not this year.

"Never eat more than you can lift." — Miss Piggy

# Damage Control
# for Holiday Eating

This holiday season, with all the opportunities to get together with family, friends and co-workers for parties and feasts, how do you avoid the temptation to overeat vast amounts of hearty food? Try these damage-control strategies:

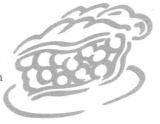

- Serve yourself with restraint: Go for small portions of rich holiday fare, while making a special effort to get hold of any vegetables and fruits in sight. The white meat of turkey is a good low-fat choice, but don't eat the fatty skin.

- Learn to say no gracefully: Notice when you feel full, and quit eating then. You don't have to take seconds — or thirds — just to prove that the food tastes delicious: If your hosts press you to eat more, why not show your delight by asking to take a portion home to share with your family.

- Take care with alcohol: Also remember to practice moderation when holiday parties offer calorie-loaded alcoholic beverages — and <u>don't</u> drink and drive.

- Cook light, lean and tasty: If you do the cooking, or plan the menu with your spouse, you can help all your guests by going easy on the fat, sugar and salt in your recipes — and serving smaller portions. Try these delicious twists on traditional favorites: bake fresh sweet potatoes instead of candying canned yams with marshmallows, or make stuffing with chestnuts and celery in place of sausage and butter.

- Start new holiday activities: Sure, it's fun to make and eat heaps of food — and to sit around a favorite holiday video, home movie or football game. And these are also ways to show that you're enjoying yourself and that you care about the people around you. But it pays to try other, less fattening, ways to have a good time and express these warm feelings: like singing or dancing together, telling stories or jokes or joining a fitness club with friends to burn off any extra calories you may have accumulated over the holidays despite your best efforts.

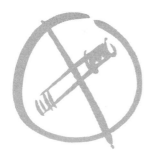

# Smoking:
# How to Kick the Habit

If you smoke, quitting is just about the healthiest thing you can do for your body. But stopping smoking can be a serious challenge. Like any addictive drug, tobacco causes withdrawal symptoms when you first kick the habit. So even though smoking-linked health risks start decreasing as soon as you quit, you may not feel your best right away.

For a few weeks after your last cigarette, you should be prepared for withdrawal symptoms such as craving for tobacco, increased appetite, nervousness and a need to find something for your mouth and hands to do. The following steps can help you overcome these symptoms — and quit for good.

## Quitting Tips

**List why you want to quit**, stressing the reasons most important to you, like "to get that bad smell out of my hair — and breath" or "so my kids won't breathe my smoke or copy my smoking." Think about why and when you smoke — like to relax with a cup of coffee. Just by analyzing your habit, you'll probably start to cut down. This tapering off should lower your body's dependence on nicotine and help you stop smoking.

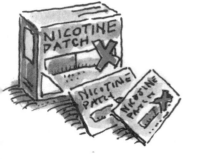

**Pick a date to give up smoking** completely, like November 15, the American Cancer Society's Great American Smokeout. Going "cold turkey" is more successful for most people. It's even better if relatives, co-workers and friends can quit on the same day — or at least not smoke around you.

**Remember, the first days are hardest:** Do whatever is needed to get through them. At first, you might have to avoid activities that trigger your urge to smoke, like hearty meals or visiting a bar. Busy your mouth and hands. Especially during the difficult early days, eat as many low-cal snacks as you want, like dried fruits, nuts, celery sticks and carrots. Chew gum — or consider a nicotine-containing gum available by prescription from your doctor or dentist. And try holding a pencil between your fingers, doodling or whittling.

**Exercise.** It will help prevent you from gaining weight, calm your nerves, reduce your urge to smoke and make you feel <u>even better</u> about all the good things you're doing for yourself simply by quitting.

**Enjoy not smoking.** Think of the healthy returns of quitting, and of all the money you're saving, and use it to treat yourself. Savor the flavor of food, now that tobacco isn't dulling your taste buds — but avoid high-calorie foods.

Most smokers who really want to stop can do it on their own. But many need the help of an individual or group counseling, hypnosis, relaxation training or behavior modification to ease withdrawal symptoms. To find a program in your area, contact the American Cancer Society, American Lung Association (see INFO-LINES at the end of this book), local hospitals or talk to your employer. And good luck!

## Fighting Nicotine with Nicotine

It's a myth that nicotine addiction is impossible to beat. The truth is, it's estimated that at least one-fifth of smokers who use nicotine replacement therapy — such as patches, gum or nasal spray — can stay smoke-free for over six months. About a third who use Zyban remain smoke-free after the same period, and results are even better when Zyban and nicotine replacement are combined. Adding behavioral counseling appears to further improve the chances of overcoming addiction.

# "It Happened So Fast!"

Automobile accidents can occur in a flash, so this holiday season, please be extra careful. If you take the time to follow these steps, you'll have miles of safe driving ahead:

A **Stay alert.** If you're tired, pull off the road to stretch or take a nap. <u>Never</u> drive when taking medicine that can make you drowsy. And if something distracts you — such as a bee buzzing inside the car — pull over to deal with it before continuing.

B **Keep control.** Slow down at night or in bad weather. And on wet roads, watch the car ahead of you especially carefully. If it isn't leaving tire tracks, it's "hydroplaning," or riding on water instead of pavement. That means the driver does not have good control. **Self-defense:** Steer clear of such vehicles.

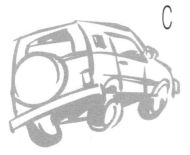

C **Cut nighttime glare. How:** Wear sunglasses for daytime driving, which makes it easier for eyes to adapt to glare at night. Keep windshields, mirrors and headlights clean, headlights aligned and eyes moving during nighttime driving. **Idea:** Consider glasses or contact lenses with anti-reflective coating, available from any optometrist or optician.

D **Ease air bag worries.** Air bags can save lives when properly used. **For maximum safety:** Sit as far from the air bag as possible and wear lap and shoulder belts. Have all children under 12 sit in the back, properly restrained. <u>Never</u> place a rear-facing infant seat in the front seat of a car with a passenger air bag.

**And of course:** Obey speed limits ... don't drink and drive ... and always keep a safe distance from the car ahead of you.

## Pull Over and Dial

Vehicle accidents while using car phones are on the rise. The *New England Journal of Medicine* reports that driving while using a cell phone is as dangerous as driving drunk! So take a few tips on talking:

- When you need to make a call, pull over, stop the car, make the call and hang up before you get back on the road. Invest in a hands-free phone.

- Don't try to take notes while driving. Remember, the fewer distractions while driving, the safer you are.

# December

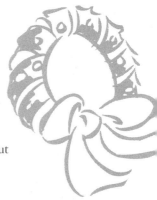

The season of giving concludes with a month filled with last minute to-dos, money-spending and get-togethers. With a reminder to be sure to take time out for yourself this month, we humbly offer up some friendly advice on how to take it easy

## 5 Secrets for a Super Holiday Season

Holidays are meant to be fun, but high expectations and hectic schedules often produce stress and anxiety. Here's how to keep this festive time of year manageable, enjoyable and relaxed:

**1** … getting ready. Create a to-do list, and then sit down with your family once a week to review progress. Delegate tasks like writing greeting cards, buying decorations or baking cookies.

**2** … shopping. Make a budget and stick to it. And if you find traffic and parking lots especially aggravating, start your shopping <u>now</u> and avoid the holiday rush. Consider shopping by catalog or online.

**3** … hosting. Try not to overplan or expect everything to be perfect. Invite only as many people as you can realistically accommodate. Use recipes that allow you to chill or freeze dishes ahead of time.

**4** … traveling. If you're flying, going by train or bus, get to the terminal or station well in advance of departure. If you're driving, leave plenty of time to arrive safely. Plan to return at least one day before you resume your normal schedule.

## Holiday Headaches?

You'll have more fun this month if you keep holiday headaches at bay.
**Prevention:** Try not to linger in smoke- or perfume-filled rooms typical of holiday celebrations, since stuffy environments can lead to headaches. And watch "party" foods like wine, cheese and processed meats. They contain amines, substances believed to trigger headache pain.

**5** ... wrapping up. Once things return to normal, take a moment to jot down what you could do differently next year as well as what went right this year. You'll sweeten the memories and get an even better handle on future celebrations.

**Plus:** Don't forget to be good to yourself, too. Get enough sleep, exercise and go easy on caffeine and alcohol. A less-stressed you could be the best gift you receive this holiday season.

*stress*

## Don't Blame the Spicy Meatball: All About Ulcers

About one in ten Americans develop ulcers, crater-like sores in the stomach or upper portion of the small intestine.

WHAT CAUSES ULCERS? Doctors used to think that ulcers were caused by stress or too much acid in the stomach. Now it's known that many ulcers are caused by a bacteria called *Helicobacter pylori* (H. *pylori*). **Fact:** It's a myth that spicy foods cause ulcers, although they may aggravate an ulcer if you have one.

OTHER CAUSES. Stress may still play a role in causing ulcers, many experts believe. Aspirin and similar pain relievers, such as ibuprofen or naproxen, can damage the protective lining of the stomach wall and also cause ulcers. **Note:** Most people with "dyspepsia" (upper abdominal pain) or stomach distress actually have gastroesophageal reflux disease (GERD). Only a doctor can tell whether you have an ulcer or GERD.

**WHAT YOU CAN DO.** Anyone with the symptoms of an ulcer — usually, burning pain on an empty stomach — should seek a doctor's treatment right away. However, you can get relief by trying the following:

- **Cut caffeine.** Coffee, cola, chocolate and other foods containing caffeine can stimulate stomach acid production.

- **Avoid alcohol.** It stimulates acid secretion and is more likely to make acid back up or "reflux" into your esophagus, giving you that sudden, burning feeling.

- **Manage stress.** Too much anxiety can upset your stomach and increase ulcer pain.

**The good news:** Eighty percent of ulcers caused by *H. pylori* can be cured with medication in two weeks ... and 80 percent of the rest can be cured with a second treatment.

## The Tree That Sneezes

**Did you know?** Some people are allergic to the molds and pollens released by their Christmas tree — especially as the tree dries out. Others are allergic to a chemical in the tree's oil.

"Health is a gift, but you have to work to keep it." — Elbert Hubbard

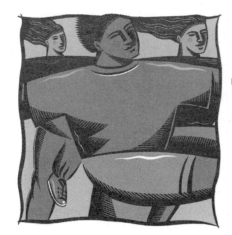

part three

TOPHEALTH
Anytime

# TopHealth Anytime

You don't have to keep your eye on the calendar to follow these timeless wellness classics. How to tone up, calm down, refuel, recharge and trim time with what you have, where you are.

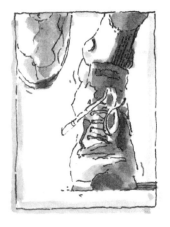

## Fast Fitness for Right Now

No time to exercise? Try these "toners" ... anytime ... anywhere.

1   Finger Flexer. Twist a rubber band around all five fingers of one hand. Gently spread your fingers wide apart against the rubber band's resistance. Relax and repeat.

2   Hamstring Curls. Stand straight, holding something stable for support (like the back of a chair). Lift one foot behind you as high as possible by bending your knee. Hold ... then lower the foot to the floor. Repeat with the other foot.

3   Leg Lifts. Sit in a chair with feet flat on the floor. Without moving your thigh, raise one foot by straightening your knee. Hold ... then bring the foot back down. Repeat with the other foot.

4   Back Stretch. Sit erect with feet apart. Place fingertips on shoulders with your elbows spread wide apart. Slowly bend over and twist so that you move one elbow across and down to the opposite knee. Straighten up and gently bring both elbows back. Repeat to the other side.

**5** Wise Walking. Building to building or office to office, take longer, quicker strides, swing your arms as you go and use stairs whenever possible. You'll boost the intensity of this "aerobic" exercise and burn more calories. **Plus:** You'll get where you're going sooner. (And you thought you didn't have time to exercise!)

"Do what you can, with what you have, where you are." — Theodore Roosevelt

## Slam the Brakes on Stressful Commutes

Traffic jams and rude drivers can sometimes make a job of getting to and from work. But there are ways to beat "stress on wheels" and enjoy the ride ...

### Get a head start.
Before leaving home or work, listen for traffic reports to avoid trouble spots. Allow for unexpected delays by leaving for work 10-15 minutes early — you'll be amazed how a little extra time can relax you. When you're able, try alternate, less congested routes like back roads or side streets.

### Compile a commuter's kit.
Equip your car with a map for escaping traffic snarls ... hard candy or sugarless gum for nerve-wracking moments ... a notepad or tape player for recording reminders when stuck in traffic. Keep relaxation tapes handy along with cassettes of soothing music, narrated books or self-improvement courses. **Idea:** Try learning another language.

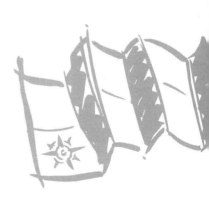

**Blow off steam.** Bottling up commuter tension can limit your ability to concentrate at work and sleep at night. So let it go. **Suggestion:** Cope with each emotional fender-bender by breathing deeply 4-5 times — from the abdomen, not the chest — to help your body defuse.

**Don't take chances.** Running yellow lights revs your motor along with your car's. Slow down, drive the speed limit and obey all rules of the road. Avoid weaving in and out of lanes to get just a few cars ahead. The measly seconds you might save aren't worth the gamble.

**Seek alternatives.** Riding buses or subways can eliminate the need to sit in bumper-to-bumper traffic and help you build more walking into your routine. And car pooling carries triple benefits: It relieves you of always having to personally deal with traffic, lets you savor the scenery and cuts your commuting costs. Now that's a "wheel" deal!

# 5 Peak Performance Boosters

Here are some of the fastest ways to condition yourself for optimum performance:

**1** **Fuel up.** Carbohydrates provide an energy boost for increased activity. So try a quick snack — banana with skim milk, whole wheat bread or a glass of orange juice — an hour or so before you want to "peak."

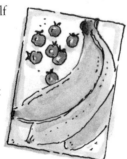

**2** Enjoy the ride. Top performers spend most of their time doing the things that lead to success, not simply "being" successful. So learn to love the journey as you tackle projects. **How:** Stop periodically to note how much you're learning, how your skills are improving, and how good you'll feel about yourself once you've accomplished the goals.

**3** Smile! Spark performance with a positive attitude. Turning the corners of your mouth upward relaxes facial muscles and then works magic on the heart rate, breathing rate and brain activity. Pretend on occasion if you have to — it still works, according to one study that found even forcing a smile produced a genuine feeling of happiness.

**4** Flip-flop "failures." Make setbacks work <u>for</u> you by seeing them as steps to success. **Examples:** If you miss a deadline, schedule extra time for the next project and if you make a mistake, realize that you've just become "smarter" and resolve not to make the same error twice. **Remember:** Failures happen and then they're over, but success goes on and on.

**5** Pile on the praise. Offer genuine compliments to colleagues for jobs well done. **Reason:** Someday they'll return the favor, making you feel like a winner and ready to tackle your next big task with renewed energy.

# Mini Meals on the Go

Our diets may not be similar, but our style of eating has something in common with cows. Even though we don't nibble on grass like our four-legged friends, we do graze on food.

Actually, there's nothing wrong with grazing, provided these "mini-meals" don't sprout a junk food farm. With forethought, snacking is an excellent way to fill in necessary calories and nutrients otherwise lacking in your diet because of incomplete or skipped meals. In fact, research shows that day-long snacking on low-fat foods can lower blood cholesterol levels even faster than eating that same food as three meals.

# Tips for low-fat, nutritious snacks

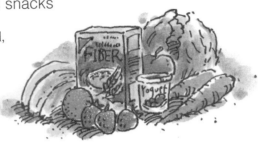

**Fruit.** Plain or delicately flavored, "nature's candy" hits the spot. Try apple slices sprinkled with cinnamon. Make melon kabobs marinated in dry white wine. Top fresh berries with nonfat yogurt.

**Vegetables.** This crunchy snack is filling, yet low in calories (about 25 per 1/2 cup), and is a generous source of the potentially cancer-protective vitamins A and C.

**Crackers.** Be selective with your choice of crackers. Crispbread (Wasa or Finn), matzo and rice cakes are lower in fat and calories than other varieties, like Ritz, Hi-Ho and Triscuit.

**Cheese.** If snacking on cheese, make sure it's the low-fat kind, such as cottage cheese made with 1 percent milk fat, farmer's cheese, or reduced-calorie cheese.

**Popcorn.** Air-popped popcorn is low in calories (only 23 per cup) and high in fiber. Avoid adding butter or margarine, which adds calories, and instead flavor with herbs or onion powder. Avoid packaged or microwave popcorn, both plain and flavored. They often contain lots of fat — and calories.

**Nuts.** Go easy on the nuts. Just 1/4 cup can have as many as 200 calories.

**Pretzels.** The next time you are staring at the vending machine deciding on a munchie, select pretzels. Ounce per ounce, they contain far less fat and calories than chips.

**Beverages.** A drink often curbs hunger and can provide needed nutrients. Low-fat milk, orange juice or vegetable juices are good choices. Happy grazing!

# 4 Ways to Beat the Clock

For more time and less stress, make the most of every minute you already have. Here's how:

TRACK your time. Audit your activities in 15- or 30-minute periods for a week. Jot down how long you spend on absolutely everything — chores, social activities and job-related tasks. You'd be surprised how much you can cut back.

LET your body clock rule. To get more done in less time, do your most challenging work in the morning, when you're most alert ... creative activities around 2 p.m., when most daydreaming occurs ... simpler tasks mid-afternoon during the post-lunch slump.

WORK while you wait. Tackle small tasks during "lost" time between meetings, standing in lines or sitting in waiting rooms. **Examples:** Read mail, start a shopping list, review project to-dos.

LIVE in the present. On average, people spend about 30 percent of their time reliving the past and another 30 percent worrying about the future. **Better:** Focus more on what's happening now. **One way:** Say out loud what you're hearing or seeing. Since you can't speak and listen to "inner voices" at the same time, you'll waste less time worrying — and immediately feel more relaxed.

# How to Get That Second Wind

Feeling run down? You'll turn things around in five minutes if you ...

1 ... REFUEL. Snack on fiber-rich munchies, such as dried apricots, bananas, baby carrots or rye wafers. **Benefit:** The fiber slows the release of glucose (a sugar) into your bloodstream and helps fight energy dips.

**2** ... BREATHE DEEPLY. Every 1-2 hours, spend five minutes inhaling and exhaling deeply, hands on ribs. You'll promote calmness and mental focus as well as renewed energy.

**3** ... GO ON AN "IMAGI-CATION."
Close your eyes and take a mental vacation by imagining a peaceful scene ... on an island ... in a meadow ... by the ocean. Imagine yourself relaxing there.

**4** ... CALL A CONFIDANTE.
Use your personal support system — family, friends or co-workers — to quickly unload and unwind.

**5** ... SNAP OUT OF IT. Splash cold water on your face, snap a rubber band worn on the wrist or pop a breath mint — mint flavors are stimulating.

**6** ... TAKE A "GOOD NEWS" INVENTORY. At the end of the day, jot down all the good things that happened. You'll be surprised at how much went right. Plus, you'll set yourself up for a good night's sleep ... and energize yourself for tomorrow.

"It takes a long time to become young." — Pablo Picasso

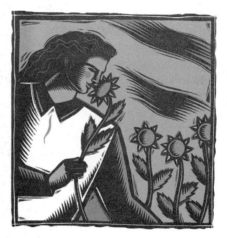

## part four

# How to Live Longer...
## Better...Happier!

# How to Live Longer ...
# Better ... Happier!

## Thoughts from Dr. Zorba's Longevity Corner

Although genetics plays a role in how many years you have left, experts say how you age is mostly a matter of how you live. From longevity expert Zorba Paster, MD, medical editor of TopHealth, here are ways to maximize your "health span" as well as your life span:

**1** **Nurture friendships.** Numerous studies have shown that people with close relationships have a lower rate of serious illness following personal crises ... while those who don't have close friends have more health problems and are unlikely to live as long.

**2** **Keep moving.**
The sooner you start exercising — even 20 minutes every other day — the lower your risk for major killers like heart disease, high blood pressure, diabetes, obesity and possibly certain types of cancer. **Idea:** Start walking with a friend.

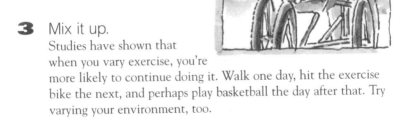

**3** **Mix it up.**
Studies have shown that when you vary exercise, you're more likely to continue doing it. Walk one day, hit the exercise bike the next, and perhaps play basketball the day after that. Try varying your environment, too.

**4** **Build strength.** Weight lifting and other strength builders combat the loss of muscle and bone that occurs as you age. **Example:** In one study, 70-year-old men were just as strong as 28-year-olds. **The difference:** The older men had done strength training since middle age; the younger men didn't strength train at all.

**5** **…But weekend warriors beware.** Recently published research in the *Journal of the American Medical Association* shows sudden intense exercise can bring on a heart attack — that is, if you're out of shape and overweight, smoke or have high cholesterol. But moderate exercise — just to the point where you break a sweat — is OK. So why not take a brisk walk over lunch? You'll boost longevity by reducing your weight and strengthening your heart.

**6** **Enjoy nature's best.** Eat a variety of whole grains, fruits and vegetables. **Benefit:** They're low in fat and calories, making it easier to achieve healthy weight and avoid major health problems like heart disease, diabetes and arthritis.

**7** **Make meals <u>magnifique</u>.** The French have half the heart attacks Americans do despite eating lots of cream, sausage and cheese. Some think it's that daily red wine, but perhaps it's the way they eat — leisurely and with gusto. So next time you sit down for dinner, take time to enjoy it. Consider topping off your meal with a small glass of red wine or grape juice. Both have flavonoids that may help protect the heart.

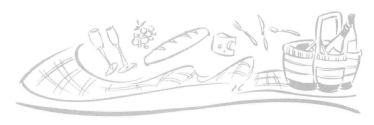

**8** **Go ahead … barbecue.** When you barbecue, the fat drips onto the coals instead of into your stomach. As fat burns it smokes the food, the taste we enjoy. But that produces nitrosamines, which some think are cancer-causing. Most scientists believe this risk is minimal. It matters more <u>what</u> you grill. Toss the hot dogs and cook lean cuts of beef — or better yet, fish and chicken. Then you can sit back and enjoy the best part about barbecuing: being with family and friends.

**9** Get regular checkups. Screening tests can detect many diseases in their early stages, when chances for successful treatment are greatest. If you haven't done so already, speak with your doctor about a screening schedule that's right for you.

**10** Think 401(k). More money when you retire means more opportunities to have the sweet life in your golden years. Important research shows that folks with a **larger** nest egg are usually healthier. **Why?** Because they have less stress. To enjoy life without the stress of financial worry: Fund your retirement plan now!

**11** Adjust your attitude. Recent research in the *British Medical Journal* shows that you can't will yourself to have cancer. But if you **do** have cancer, the right attitude will keep you alive longer and make you healthier and happier. Research on terminal breast cancer patients has shown that women who have family support and go to cancer support groups are more likely to enjoy the life they have left — and live longer.

**12** Avoid the high cost of hostility. A recent study of 18- to 30-year-olds shows that if you're a hostile young adult you may end up with a premature heart attack. There are many antidotes to hostility, such as counseling, meditation and avoiding intoxicants. Antidepressants often work, as many hostile people are depressed. But our favorite is volunteerism: The act of giving uplifts the spirit and can add years to your longevity.

**13** Pursue pleasures. Consider "can't-hurt-could-help" strategies to help enjoy the passage of time. **Suggestions:** Try a sauna occasionally ... practice daily meditation ... make time for music and art ... bring flowers into your home.

**14** Take the vacation prescription. According to recent research, men who take vacations live longer than those who don't. A yearly vacation appears to cut risk of a deadly heart attack by more than 33 percent. Vacations are a time to relax, have fun, ponder what life's about. When you resume everyday life, you often have more zest and increase your longevity.

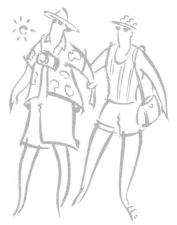

**15** Adjust your attitude. Seriously ... laughing eases tension, improves circulation, boosts alertness and helps strengthen relationships. So see a comedy play, read a humor magazine and exchange funny stories with a friend — and laugh your whole life long.

*Dr. Zorba Paster is a Clinical Professor of Family Medicine and is on the Board of Directors of the Wisconsin Academy of Family Physicians. Dr. Paster is also a television Medical News Commentator and his radio program, "Zorba Paster on Your Health" is heard by countless health- and fitness-conscious listeners on National Public Radio. Look for his newest book, <u>The Longevity Code: Your Personal Prescription for a Longer Sweeter Life</u>, available February 2001.*

"May you live all the days of your life." — Jonathan Swift

# Where to Find
# Free Health Information

The following organizations offer free information; many will also send free publications upon request. You may also call the National Health Information Center (800-336-4797) for information or referral to an organization that can help you with your questions. If you don't have access to the Internet, try your local library.

## Alcohol

National Clearinghouse for Alcohol and Drug Information
800-729-6686
www.health.org

American Council on Alcoholism
800-527-5344

## Allergies and Asthma

Allergy and Asthma Network
800-878-4403
www.aanma.org

American College of Allergy, Asthma and Immunology
800-822-2762
www.aaaai.org

## Cancer Prevention
## and Management

American Cancer Society
800-227-2345
www.cancer.org/
National Cancer Institute
800-4-CANCER (422-6237)
www.nih.nci.gov

# Consumer Issues/Health

American Institute for Preventive Medicine
800-345-2476
www.aipm.healthy.net

# Depression

National Institute of Mental Health
800-421-4211.
www.nimh.nih.gov

# Diabetes

American Diabetes Association
800-232-3472
www.diabetes.org

# Ears and Hearing

Better Hearing Institute-Hearing Help Line
800-327-9355

# Eye Health and Safety

American Optometric Association
314-991-4100
www.aoa.net

Prevent Blindness America
800-331-2020
www.preventblindness.org

# Family Health

American Academy of Family Physicians
www.familydoctor.org

## Food Safety

USDA Meat and Poultry Hotline
800-535-4555

## Headaches

National Headache Foundation
800-843-2256
www.headaches.org

## Glaucoma

Prevent Blindness America
800-331-2020
www.preventblindness.org

## Heart Health

American Heart Association
800-242-8721
www.amhrt.org

National Heart, Lung and Blood Institute
800-575-9355 (WELL)
www.nhlbi.nih.gov

## Nutrition and Weight Control

American Dietetic Association
800-366-1655
www.eatright.org

## Osteoporosis

National Osteoporosis Foundation
800-223-9994
www.nof.org

## Poison Prevention

Pharmacist Planning Services, Inc.
415-479-8628
E-mail: ppsi@aol.com

## Sleep

National Sleep Foundation
888-673-7533
www.sleepfoundation.org

## Smoking Cessation

Great American Smokeout
American Cancer Society
800-227-2345
www.cancer.org

American Lung Association
800-LUNG-USA (586-4872)
www.lungusa.org

## NOTE
You can find hundreds of toll-free health information hotlines
in the National Library of Medicine's "Health Hotlines" database.
Just go to sis.nlm.nih.gov/hotlines.

infolines

# Resource & Contact List

## Administration on Aging

200 Independence Avenue SW
Washington, DC 20201
(202)401–4541
www.aoa.gov

## Advocates for Youth

1025 Vermont Avenue NW, Suite 200
Washington, DC 20005
(202)347-5700
info@advocatesforyouth.org
www.advocatesforyouth.org

## Alzheimer's Disease
## and Related Disorders Association

919 North Michigan Avenue, Suite 1100
Chicago, IL 60611–1676
(800)272–3900
(312)335–8882 (TDD)

## American Academy of Dermatology

P.O. Box 4014
Schaumburg, IL 60168
(847)330–0230 ext. 343
www.aad.org

## American Academy of Family Physicians

8880 Ward Parkway
Kansas City, MO 64114–2797
(800)274–2237
www.aafp.org

## American Academy of Ophthalmology

P.O. Box 7242
San Francisco, CA 94120-7424
(415)561-8500
(415)561-8567 (Fax)
www.evenet.org

## American Academy of Pediatrics

141 Northwest Point Boulevard
Elk Grove Village, IL 60007
(847)981–7667
(847)981–7134 (message line)
www.aap.org

## American Association of Cardiovascular and Pulmonary Rehabilitation

7611 Elmwood Avenue, Suite 201
Middleton, WI 53562
(608)831–6989
aacvpr@tmahq.com
www.aacvpr.org

## American Association for World Health

1825 K Street NW, Suite 1208
Washington, DC 20006
(202)466–5883
AAWHstaff@aol.com


## American Association of Suicidology

4201 Connecticut Avenue N., Suite 310
Washington, DC 20008
(202)237–2280
www.suicidology.org


## American Cancer Society

1599 Clifton Road NE
Atlanta, GA 30329–4251
(800)ACS–2345
www.cancer.org


## American Chiropractic Association

1701 Clarendon Boulevard
Arlington, VA 22209
(703)276–8800
AmerChiro@aol.com
www.amerchiro.org


## American Counseling Association

5999 Stevenson Avenue
Alexandria, VA 22304
(703)823–9800
aca@counseling.org
www.counseling.org

# American Dental Association

211 E. Chicago Avenue
Chicago, IL 60611
(800)947-4746; (800)621-8099
www.ada.org

# American Dental Hygienists Association

444 North Michigan Avenue, Suite 3400
Chicago, IL 60611
(312)440-8900
www.adha.org

# American Diabetes Association

1660 Duke Street
Alexandria, VA 22314
(800)232-3472
www.diabetes.org

# American Dietetic Association

216 West Jackson Boulevard
Suite 800
Chicago, IL 60606-6995
(312)899-0040
www.eatright.org

# American Heart Association

7272 Greenville Avenue
Dallas, TX 75231
(800)AHA-USA1
inquire@amhrt.org
www.americanheart.org

## American Institute for Preventive Medicine

30445 Northwestern Highway, Suite 350
Farmington Hills, MI 48334
(248)539–1800, ext. 247
aipm.healthy.net


## American Liver Foundation

1425 Pompton Avenue
Cedar Grove, NJ 07009
(800)GO–LIVER
www.liverfoundation.org


## American Lung Association

1740 Broadway
New York, NY 10019–4374
(800)LUNG–USA
info@lunusa.org
www.lungusa.org


## The American Occupational Therapy Association, Inc.

4720 Montgomery Lane, Box 31220
Bethesda, MD 20824–1220
(301)652–2682
praoto@aota.org
www.aota.org


## American Optometric Association

243 North Lindbergh Boulevard
St. Louis, MO 63141
(314)991–4100
www.aoanet.org

## American Physical Therapy Association

1111 North Fairfax Street
Alexandria, VA 22314
(703)706–3248 x3248
www.apta.org

## American Psychiatric Association

1400 K Street NW
Washington, DC 20005
(202)682–6220
www.psych.org

## American Public Health Association

800 Eye Street NW
Washington, DC 20005
(202)777–APHA
www.apha.org

## American Social Health Association

P.O. Box 13827
Research Triangle Park, NC 27709
(919)361–8400
www.ashastd.org

## American Speech-Language-Hearing Association

10801 Rockville Pike
Rockville, MD 20852
(800)638–8255
irc@asha.org
www.asha.org

## American Trauma Society

8903 Presidential Parkway, Suite 512
Upper Marlboro, MD 20772–2656
(800)556–7890
atstrauma@aol.com
www.amtrauma.org

## Aplastic Anemia Foundation of America, Inc.

P.O. Box 613
Annapolis, MD 21404
(800)747–2820
afacenter@aol.com
www.aplastic.org

## The Arc

500 East Border Street, Suite 300
Arlington, TX 76010
(817)261–6003
www.thearc.org

## Association for the Care of Children's Health

19 Mantua Road
Mount Royal, NJ 08061
(609)224–1742
www.acch.org

## Asthma and Allergy Foundation of America

1233 20th Street NW, Suite 402
Washington, DC 20036
(800)7–ASTHMA
info@aafa.org
www.aafa.org

## Autism Society of America

7910 Woodmont Avenue, Suite 300
Bethesda, MD 20814–3015
(800)3–AUTISM (parent information and referral calls only)
(800)329–0899 (fax-on demand, quick response)
www.autism-society.org/asa/home.html

## Campaign for Tobacco-Free Kid's National Action Network

(800)284–KIDS
www.tobaccofreekids.org

## Cancer Research Foundation of America

1600 Duke Street, Suite 110
Alexandria, VA 22314
(800) 227-CRFA
(703)836-4412
www.preventcancer.org

## Centers for Disease Control and Prevention

National Immunization Program
1600 Clifton Road, Mail Stop E52
Atlanta, GA 30333
(800)232–2522 (English)
(800)232–0233 (Spanish)
www.cdc.gov/nip

resource & contact list

## Dana Alliance for Brain Initiatives

745 Fifth Avenue, Suite 200
New York, NY 10151
(212)223-4040
dabiinfo@dana.org
www.dana.org/dabi/dabi.html

## Educational Television Network, Inc.

P.O. Box 7536
Wilton, CN 06897
(203)834–9888
(203)762–0207 (Fax)
healthyaging.net

## Epilepsy Foundation of America

4351 Garden City Drive
Landover, MD 20785
(800)EFA–1000
(800)213–5821 (Publications)
www.efa.org

## Eye Bank Association of America

1015 18th Street NW, Suite 1010
Washington, DC 20036
(202)775–4999
sightebaa@aol.com
www.restoresight.org

## Families of Spinal Muscular Atrophy

P.O. Box 196
Libertyville, IL 60048-0196
(800)886-1762
sma@interaccess.com
www.fsma.org

## Food Allergy Network

10400 Eaton Place, Suite 107
Fairfax, VA 22030-2208
(703)691-3179
FAN@worldweb.net
www.foodallergy.org

## Gynecologic Cancer Foundation

401 N. Michigan Avenue
Chicago, IL 60611
(800)444-4441
(312) 644-6610
gcf@sba.com
www.wcn.org

## Health Information Resource Center

621 East Park Avenue
Libertyville, IL 60048-2904
(800)828-8225
hlthinfo@aol.com
www.nahdo.org/nhirc/index.html

resource & contact list

## Healthy Weight Network

402 South 14th Street
Hettinger, ND 58639
(701)567-2646


## Helen Keller National Center

111 Middle Neck Road
Sands Point, NY 11050
(516)944-8900, ext. 325
(516)944-8637 (TTY)
HKncpr@aol.com
www.helenkeller.org


## Hemochromatosis Foundation

P.O. Box 8569
Albany, NY 12208
(518)489-0972
www.hemochromatosis.org


## Hepatitis Foundation International

30 Sunrise Terrace
Cedar Grove, NJ 07009
(973)239-1035
HFI@intac.com
www.hepfi.org


## International Food Safety Council

(312)715-0807
www.foodsafetycouncil.org

# Juvenile Products Manufacturers Association

236 Route 38-West, Suite 100
Moorestown, NJ 08057
www.jpma.org


# Lupus Foundation of America

1300 Piccard Drive, Suite 200
Rockville, MD 20850–4303
(800)558–0121
www.lupus.org


# March of Dimes Birth Defects Foundation

1275 Mamaroneck Avenue
White Plains, NY 10605
(888)MODIMES
www.modimes.org


# National Cancer Institute/Better Health Foundation

6130 Executive Boulevard, EPN 232
Bethesda, MD 20892-7332
(301)496-8520
www.nci.nig.gov


# National Cervical Cancer Coalition

16501 Sherman Way Avenue
Suite 110
Van Nuys, CA 91406
(818)909-3849
(818)780-8199 (Fax)
ncccak@nccc-online.org
www.nccc-online.org

## National Coalition Against Domestic Violence

6400 Flank Drive, Suite 1300
Harrisburg, PA 17112-2778
(800)799–7233
(303)839–1852
www.ncadv.org

## National Coalition for Adult Immunization

4733 Bethesda Avenue, Suite 750
Bethesda, MD 20814–5228
(301)656–0003
www.nfid.org/ncai

## National Center for Health Education

72 Spring Street, Suite 208
New York, NY 10012
(212)334–9470 ext. 0
www.nche.org

## National Chronic Fatigue Syndrome and Fibromyalgia Association

P.O. Box 18426
Kansas City, MO 64133
(816)313–2000

## National Committee to Prevent Child Abuse

200 South Michigan Avenue
Suite 1700
Chicago, IL 60604
(312)663–3520
www.parentsoup.com/library/organizations/bpd0325.html

## National Council for Adoption

1930 17th Street NW
Washington, DC 20009
(202)328–1200
info@ncfa-usa.org
www.ncfa-usa.org

## National Council on Alcoholism and Drug Dependence, Inc.

12 West 21st Street, Seventh floor
New York, NY 10010
(212)206–6770
National@NCADD.org
www.ncadd.org

## National Council on Patient Information and Education

4915 St. Elmo Avenue, Suite 505
Bethesda, MD 20814-6053
(301)656–8565
(301)656–4464 (Fax)
ncpie@erols.com
www.talkaboutrx.org

## National Fire Protection Association

P.O. Box 9101
1 Batterymarch Park
Quincy, MA 02269
(800)344–3555 (orders only)
custserv@NFPA.org
www.nfpa.org

## National Headache Foundation (NHF)

428 West St. James Place, 2nd Floor
Chicago, IL 60614–2750
(800)843–2256
www.headaches.org


## National Heart, Lung, and Blood Institute Information Center

P.O. Box 30105
Bethesda, MD 20824–0105
(301)592–8573
(301)592–8563 (Fax)
nhlbiinfo@rover.nhlbi.nih.gov
www.nhlbi.nih.gov


## National Hemophilia Foundation

116 West 32nd Street, 11th Floor
New York, NY 10001
(800)42–HANDI
info@hemophilia.org
www.hemophilia.org


## National Highway Transportation Safety Administration

U.S. Department of Transportation
400 Seventh Street SW
Washington, DC 20590
(202)366–9550
www.nhtsa.dot.gov

## National Kidney Foundation

30 East 33rd Street
New York, NY 10016
(800)622–9010
www.kidney.org

## National Inhalant Prevention Coalition

2904 Kirby Lane
Austin, TX 78703
(800)269–4237
www.inhalants.org

## National Marrow Donor Program®

3433 Broadway Street NE, Suite 500
Minneapolis, MN 55413
(800)627–7692
www.marrow.org

## National Men's Health Week

14 East Minor Street
Emmaus, PA 18098
(610)967–8620
www.nationalmenshealthweek.com

## National Mental Health Association

1021 Prince Street
Alexandria, VA 22314–2971
(800)969–6642
www.nmha.org

## National Osteoporosis Foundation

1232 22nd Street NW
Washington, DC 20037
(202)223–2226
www.nof.org


## National Rehabilitation Awareness Foundation

P.O. Box 71
Scranton, PA 18501–0071
(717)341–4637
www.allied-services.org


## National Reye's Syndrome Foundation

P.O. Box 829
Bryan, OH 43506
(419)636–2679
reyessyn@mail.bright.net
www.bright.net/~reyessyn


## National SAFE KIDS Campaign

1301 Pennsylvania Avenue NW, Suite 1000
Washington, DC 20004–1707
(202)662–0600
info@safekids.org
www.safekids.org

## National Safety Council
(Partnership for a Walkable America)

1121 Spring Lake Drive
Itasca, IL 60143-3201
(630)775-2185 (Fax)
thompsoh@nsc.org
www.nsc.org/walkable.htm


## National Stroke Association

96 Inverness Drive, East, Suite 1
Englewood, CO 80112–5112
(800)STROKES
www.stroke.org


## National Therapeutic Recreation Society

National Recreation and Park Association
22377 Belmont Ridge Road
Ashburn, VA 20148
(703)858–0784
NTRSNRPA@aol.com
www.nrpa.org/branches/ntrs.html


## National Youth Sports Safety Foundation

333 Longwood Avenue, Suite 202
Boston, MA 02115
(617)277–1171
NYSSF@aol.com
www.nyssf.org

## Office of Occupant Protection

National Highway Traffic Safety Administration
U.S. Department of Transportation
400 Seventh Street SW
Washington, DC 20590
(202)366–9550
www.nhtsa.dot.gov


## Planned Parenthood Federation of America

810 Seventh Avenue
New York, NY 10019
(212)261–4628
communications@ppfa.org
www.plannedparenthood.org


## Poison Prevention Week Council

P.O. Box 1543
Washington, DC 20013
(301)504-0580 ext. 1184
www.cpsc.gov


## Prevent Blindness America

500 East Remington Road
Schaumburg, IL 60173
(800)331–2020
www.preventblindness.org

## School Food Service Association

1600 Duke Street, Seventh Floor
Alexandria, VA 22314
(800)877–8822
asfsa@asfsa.org
www.asfsa.org

## Scleroderma Foundation

89 Newbury Street, Suite 201
Danvers, MA 01923
(800)722–HOPE
sfinfo@scleroderma.org

## Shriners Burn Institute

3229 Burnet Avenue
Cincinnati, OH 45229
(513)872–6000
shriners.com/hospitals

## Sickle Cell Disease Association of America, Inc.

200 Corporate Pointe, Suite 495
Culver City, CA 90230–7633
(800)421–8453
SickleCellDisease.org

## SIDS Alliance

1314 Bedford Avenue, Suite 210
Baltimore, MD 21208
(800)221–SIDS
sidshq@charm.ne
www.sidsalliance.org

## 3D Prevention Month Coalition

1900 L Street NW, Suite 705
Washington, DC 20036
(202)452–6004


## United States Department of Health and Human Services

Health Resources and Services Adm.
Maternal and Child Health Bureau
Parklawn Building, Room 18-20
5600 Fishers Lane
Rockville, MD 20857
(301)443–0205
pcampbell@hrsa.dhhs.gov
www.mchb.hrsa.gov


## United States Eye Injury Registry (USEIR)

Box 55565
Birmingham, AL 35255
(205)933–0064


## Women's Sports Foundation

Eisenhower Park
East Meadow, NY 11554
(516)542–4700
wosport@aol.com
www.womenssportsfoundation.org

## World Alliance for Breastfeeding Action and La Leche League International

1400 North Meacham Road
Schaumburg, IL 60173-4840
(847)519–7730
www.lalecheleague.org

## YMCA of the USA

101 North Wacker Drive
Chicago, IL 60606
(312)269–1198
www.ymca.net

_____

_____

_____

_____

_____

_____

_____

_____

_____

_____

_____

_____

_____

_____

_____

_____

notes

_____

_____

_____

_____

_____

_____

_____

_____

_____

_____

_____

_____

_____

_____

_____

_____

To Order
Additional
Copies of:

# TOPHEALTH

## almanac
## 2001

## ☑ Yes!

Rush me additional copies
of TOPHEALTH Almanac 2001.

*Residents of Alabama, please add 4% sales tax.
Shipping and handling will be billed separately.

**MAIL** order to:
**TOPHEALTH ALMANAC 2001**
P.O. Box 381116,
Birmingham, AL 35238-1116

**FAX** to: (205) 991-2870
**TEL**: (800) 871-9525

---

## Money-Back
## Guarantee

If you or your organization is not
totally satisfied with TOPHEALTH
Almanac 2001, simply return the
almanacs and we will refund
your payment in full.

---

*Great Stocking Stuffers for
Family and Friends!*

---

## TOPHEALTH ALMANAC 2001

| | | |
|---|---|---|
| Number of copies | X | ___ |
| Price per copy | $ | 8.95 |
| | = $ | ___ |

Name
_____

Title
_____

Company
_____

Street Address
_____

_____

City
_____

State, Zip
_____

Phone
_____

Fax
_____

E-mail Address
_____

❑ Please bill me. Charge my:
   ❑ VISA    ❑ MasterCard
   ❑ NOVUS/Discover  ❑ American Express

_____
Account No.

_____
Exp. Date

_____
Signature

Priority Code: 00Y003

For discounted bulk pricing, please call
toll-free 800.871.9525.